Advance praise for *The Diabetes Code*

"By understanding the underlying cause of the disease, Dr. Fung reveals how [type 2 diabetes] can be prevented and also reversed using natural dietary methods instead of medications. This is an important and timely book. Highly recommended."

MARK HYMAN, MD, author of *Food: What the Heck Should I Eat?*

"With rich scientific support, Dr. Jason Fung has sounded a clarion call to re-evaluate how we view and treat diabetes. Considering that roughly half of all adults worldwide are diabetic or on their way (pre-diabetes), *The Diabetes Code* is essential reading."

DR. BENJAMIN BIKMAN, Associate Professor of Physiology, Brigham Young University

"In *The Diabetes Code*, Dr. Fung lays out the case for eliminating sugar and refined carbohydrates and replacing them with whole foods with healthy fats. Dr. Fung gives an easy-to-follow solution to reversing type 2 diabetes by addressing the root cause, diet."

MARIA EMMERICH, author of *The 30-Day Ketogenic Cleanse*

"In this terrific and hopeful book, Dr. Fung teaches you everything you need to know about how to reverse type 2 diabetes. It could change the world."

DR. ANDREAS EENFELDT, author of *Low Carb, High Fat Food Revolution*

"*The Diabetes Code* should be on the bookshelf of every physician and any patient struggling with blood sugar control."

CARRIE DIULUS, MD, medical director of the Crystal Clinic Spine Wellness Center

"*The Diabetes Code* is unabashedly provocative yet practical . . . a clear blueprint for everyone to take control of their blood sugar, their health, and their lives."

DR. WILL COLE, leading functional medicine practitioner and educator at drwillcole.com

"With his trademark humor, Jason Fung exposes the secret that type 2 diabetes can be reversed with the right combination of diet and lifestyle—you can reclaim your health and vitality. Dr. Fung will teach you how."

AMY BERGER, MS, CNS, author of *The Alzheimer's Antidote*

"*The Diabetes Code* clears the fog around type 2 diabetes and underscores that for most people, it is preventable or reversible."

DR. KARIM KHAN, MD, *British Journal of Sports Medicine*

DR. JASON FUNG

foreword by **NINA TEICHOLZ**

THE
DIABETES
CODE

PREVENT AND REVERSE TYPE 2 DIABETES NATURALLY

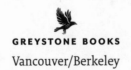

GREYSTONE BOOKS
Vancouver/Berkeley

Greystone Books Ltd.
www.greystonebooks.com

Cataloguing data available from Library and Archives Canada
ISBN 978-1-77164-265-1 (pbk.)
ISBN 978-1-77164-266-8 (epub)

Editing by Lucy Kenward
Copy editing by Lynne Melcombe
Cover and text design by Nayeli Jimenez
Printed and bound in Canada on ancient-forest-friendly paper by Friesens.

We gratefully acknowledge the support of the Canada Council for the Arts, the British
Columbia Arts Council, the Province of British Columbia through the Book Publishing
Tax Credit, and the Government of Canada for our publishing activities.

Canadä

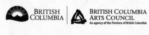

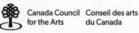

I would like to dedicate this book to my beautiful wife, Mina.
You are my guiding star, without which I would be forever lost.
You are my life, my love, my everything.

CONTENTS

....

Part 5: How to Effectively Treat Type 2 Diabetes

FOREWORD

....

I N JUST A generation, diabetes has gone from rarity to epidemic, a
catastrophic turn that presents urgent questions: Why are so many
suffering, and so suddenly? And how have our health authorities
failed to offer an explanation or treatment for so devastating a scourge,
despite spending billions? They have, instead, essentially given up on
finding a cure, pronouncing type 2 diabetes[1] a chronic, progressive disease that promises a life of slow, painful decline and early death.

Tragically, diabetes authorities worldwide have come to the consensus that the best hope for sufferers is merely to control or delay the
disease through a lifelong dependence on medications combined with
medical devices and surgery. There is no emphasis on better nutrition.
Instead, some forty-five international medical and scientific societies
and associations around the world declared in 2016 that bariatric surgery, which is both expensive and risky, should be the first option for
diabetes treatment. Another recently approved idea is a new weight-
loss procedure in which a thin tube, implanted in the stomach, ejects
food from the body before all the calories can be absorbed, which some
have termed "medically sanctioned bulimia." And all this is in addition to the basic regimen for diabetes sufferers: multiple medications,
which cost hundreds of dollars a month, and which include insulin, a
drug that paradoxically often causes weight *gain*.

These techniques for managing diabetes are expensive, invasive, and do nothing to reverse diabetes—because, as Dr. Jason Fung explains in *The Diabetes Code*, "you can't use drugs [or devices] to cure a dietary disease."

The groundbreaking idea Dr. Fung presents in these pages is that diabetes is caused by our bodies' insulin response to chronic overconsumption of carbohydrates and that the best and most natural way to reverse the disease is to reduce consumption of those carbohydrates. A low-carbohydrate diet for treating obesity is not only being practiced now by hundreds of doctors around the world but is supported by more than seventy-five clinical trials, conducted on altogether thousands of people, including several trials of two years' duration, which establish the diet as safe and effective.

Remarkably, the practice of carbohydrate restriction for diabetes dates back more than a century, when the diet was considered standard treatment. According to a 1923 medical text by the "father of modern medicine," Sir William Osler, the disease could be defined as one in which "the normal utilization of carbohydrate is impaired." Yet soon thereafter, when pharmaceutical insulin became available, that advice changed, allowing a higher-carbohydrate intake to again become the norm.

Osler's idea would not be revived until science journalist Gary Taubes unearthed and developed it into a comprehensive intellectual framework for the "carbohydrate-insulin" hypothesis, in his seminal 2007 book *Good Calories, Bad Calories*. And the modern-day clinical model for diabetics was set forth by scientists Stephen D. Phinney and Jeff S. Volek, as well as the physician Richard K. Bernstein.[2]

In an exciting recent development, clinical trial evidence specifically on diabetics is now emerging. As of this writing, at least one trial, involving some 330 people, is underway for the treatment of the disease with a very low-carbohydrate diet. At the one-year mark, researchers found that some 97 percent of patients had reduced or halted their insulin use, and 58 percent no longer had a formal diagnosis of diabetes.[3] In other words, these patients successfully reversed their diabetes simply by restricting carbohydrates—findings that ought to be compared to the official standard of care for diabetics, which states with 100 percent certainty that the condition is "irreversible."

Dr. Fung, a practicing nephrologist who gained renown by introducing intermittent fasting for the control of obesity, is a passionate and articulate proponent of the low-carbohydrate approach. In addition to his fascinating insights, he has a gift for explaining complex science clearly and delivering it with the perfect, telling anecdote. One never forgets, for instance, the image of Japanese rush-hour commuters being shoved into overstuffed subways cars as a metaphor for excessive circulating glucose packed into each and every corporeal cell. We get the point: the body cannot handle so much glucose! Dr. Fung explains the relationship between glucose and insulin and how these together drive not only obesity and diabetes but also, quite likely, a host of other related chronic diseases as well.

The obvious question is why this low-carbohydrate approach is not more widely known. Indeed, in the six months prior to my writing this foreword, major review articles on obesity appeared in such respected publications as the *New York Times, Scientific American,* and *Time* magazine, yet among the thousands of words written, there was barely a mention of the word that can explain so much: insulin. This oversight is perplexing but is also, unfortunately, the reflection of genuine bias pervading an expert community that has for half a century endorsed a very different approach.

That approach, of course, has been to count calories and avoid fat. In recent years, authorities including the U.S. Department of Agriculture and Department of Health and Human Services, which jointly publish *Dietary Guidelines for Americans,* as well as the American Heart Association, have backed off the "low-fat" diet, yet they still believe weight control can be explained by little more than a model of Calories In, Calories Out. A good deal of rigorous science debunks this notion, and the epidemics of chronic disease have not, to date, been curbed by it, but its captivating simplicity and widespread expert support allow it to endure.

There is also the stark reality that most medical associations today are significantly funded by pharmaceutical and device companies, which have no interest in a dietary solution to disease. Indeed, a nutritional fix that reverses disease and ends the need for medication puts them squarely out of business. This must explain why attendees at recent annual meetings of the American Diabetes Association (ADA) have reported that amidst a sea of presentations on medical devices and surgeries, there's a near-complete absence of any information on low-carbohydrate diets. And this fact must explain why, when the medical directors of two obesity clinics (including one at Harvard University) wrote an op-ed published in the *New York Times* about the lack of discussion on diet at the 2016 ADA conference, the ADA itself shot them down.[4] One might assume also that, in addition to financial conflicts of interest, the cognitive dissonance must be overwhelming for experts confronting information implying that their knowledge and advice of the past fifty years is simply wrong. In fact, more than wrong: harmful.

For this is the unvarnished truth: the success of carbohydrate restriction directly implies that the last several decades of low-fat, *high*-carbohydrate nutrition advice has almost certainly fueled the very obesity and diabetes epidemics it was intended to prevent. This is a devastating conclusion to half a century of public health efforts, but if we are to have any hope of reversing these epidemics, we must accept this possibility, begin to explore the alternative science contained in this book, and start on a new path forward—for the sake of truth, science, and better health.

NINA TEICHOLZ
Author of the international bestseller, *The Big Fat Surprise* (Simon & Schuster 2014)

HOW TO REVERSE AND PREVENT TYPE 2 DIABETES: THE QUICK START GUIDE

....

THIRTY YEARS AGO, home electronics, such as a brand new VCR, came with a thick instruction manual. "Read thoroughly before proceeding," it implored, and then launched into detailed setup procedures and troubleshooting guides that painstakingly described everything that could possibly go wrong. Most of us ignored this manual, plugged in our new purchase, and then tried to figure out the rest when the time clock began to blink 12:00.

Today, new electronics come with a quick start guide that outlines a few basic steps to get your machine working. Everything else is still referenced in a detailed instruction manual, now often found online, but there's really no need to consult it until you want your machine to perform more complex functions. Instruction manuals are just so much more useful this way.

Consider this section of the book the quick start guide for reversing and preventing type 2 diabetes. It's a brief introduction to the disease: what it is, why conventional treatment approaches don't work, and what you can do today to start effectively managing your health.

FACT: TYPE 2 DIABETES IS FULLY
REVERSIBLE AND PREVENTABLE

MOST HEALTH PROFESSIONALS consider type 2 diabetes to be a chronic and progressive disease. This promotes the idea that type 2 diabetes is a one-way street, a life sentence with no possibility of parole: the disease continually gets worse until you eventually require insulin injections.

But this is actually a great big lie, which is excellent news for anyone who has been diagnosed with prediabetes or type 2 diabetes. Recognizing the fallacy of this belief is the crucial first step in reversing the disease. Actually, most people already instinctively recognize this. It's ridiculously easy to prove that type 2 diabetes is almost always reversible.

Suppose you have a friend who is diagnosed with type 2 diabetes, meaning the level of glucose in his blood is continuously above normal levels. He works hard to lose 50 pounds, which enables him to stop taking his glucose-lowering medications because the levels in his blood are now normal. What would you say to him? Probably something like "Great job. You're really taking care of yourself. Keep it up!"

What you *wouldn't* say is something like "You're such a filthy liar. My doctor says this is a chronic and progressive disease so you must be lying." It seems perfectly obvious that the diabetes reversed because your friend lost all that weight. And that's the point: *type 2 diabetes is a reversible disease.*

We've intuitively sensed this truth all along. But only diet and lifestyle changes—*not* medications—will reverse this disease, simply because type 2 diabetes is largely a dietary disease. The most important determinant, of course, is weight loss. Most of the medications used to treat type 2 diabetes do not cause weight loss. Quite the contrary. Insulin, for example, is notorious for causing weight *gain*. Once patients start on insulin injections for type 2 diabetes, they often sense they are heading down the wrong path.

My diabetic patients would often say, "Doctor, you've always said weight loss is the key to reversing diabetes. Yet you prescribed me a drug that made me gain 25 pounds. How is that good?" I never had a satisfactory answer to this important question because none existed. The plain truth was that it was *not* good. The key to treating diabetes properly was weight loss. Logically, because it caused weight gain, insulin was not making things better; it was actually making the disease worse.

Since weight loss is the key to reversing type 2 diabetes, medications don't help. We only pretend they do, which is the reason most doctors think type 2 diabetes is chronic and progressive. We've avoided facing an inconvenient truth: *drugs won't cure a dietary disease.* They are about as useful as bringing a snorkel to a bicycle race. The problem is not the disease; the problem is the way we treat the disease.

The same principles used for reversing type 2 diabetes also apply to preventing it. Obesity and type 2 diabetes are closely related, and generally, increased weight increases the risk of disease. The correlation is not perfect but, nevertheless, maintaining an ideal weight is a first step to prevention.

Many people paint type 2 diabetes as an inevitable part of modern life, but this is simply not true. The epidemic of type 2 diabetes really only started in the late 1980s. So we only need to go back a single generation to find a way of life that can prevent most incidents of this disease.

FACT: TYPE 2 DIABETES IS CAUSED BY TOO MUCH SUGAR

AT ITS VERY core, type 2 diabetes can be understood as a disease caused by too much insulin, which our bodies secrete when we eat too much sugar. Framing the problem this way is incredibly powerful because the solution becomes immediately obvious. We must lower our insulin levels by reducing our dietary intake of sugar and refined carbohydrates (a form of sugar).

Imagine your body as a big sugar bowl. At birth, the bowl is empty. Over several decades, you eat sugar and refined carbohydrates and the bowl gradually fills up. When you next eat, sugar comes in and spills over the sides of the bowl because the bowl is already full.

The same situation exists in your body. When you eat sugar, your body secretes the hormone insulin to help move the sugar into your cells, where it's used for energy. If you don't burn off that sugar sufficiently, then over decades your cells become completely filled and cannot handle any more. The next time you eat sugar, insulin cannot force any more of it into your overflowing cells, so it spills out into the blood. Sugar travels in your blood in a form called glucose, and having too much of it—known as high blood glucose—is a primary symptom of type 2 diabetes.

When there's too much glucose in the blood, insulin does not appear to be doing its usual job of moving the sugar into the cells. We then say that the body has become insulin resistant, but it's not truly insulin's fault. The primary problem is that the cells are overflowing with glucose. The high blood glucose is only part of the issue. Not only is there too much glucose in the blood, there's too much glucose in all of the cells. Type 2 diabetes is simply an overflow phenomenon that occurs when there is too much glucose in *the entire body*.

In response to excess glucose in the blood, the body secretes even more insulin to overcome this resistance. This forces more glucose into the overflowing cells to keep blood levels normal. This works, but the effect is only temporary because it has not addressed the problem of excess sugar; it has only moved the excess from the blood to the cells, making insulin resistance worse. At some point, even with more insulin, the body cannot force any more glucose into the cells.

Think about packing a suitcase. At first, the clothes go into the empty suitcase without any trouble. Once the suitcase is full, however, it becomes difficult to jam in those last two T-shirts. You reach a point where you can't close the suitcase. You could say the luggage appears to be resisting the clothes. This is similar to the overflow phenomenon we see in our cells.

Once that suitcase is full, you might simply use more force to shove those last T-shirts in. This strategy will only work temporarily, because you have not addressed the underlying problem of the overfilled suitcase. As you force more shirts into the suitcase, the problem—let's call it luggage resistance—only becomes worse. The better solution is to remove some of the clothes from the suitcase.

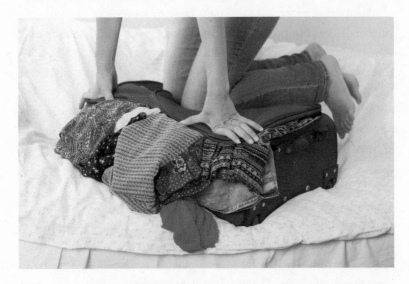

What happens in the body if we do not remove the excess glucose? First, the body keeps increasing the amount of insulin it produces to try to force more glucose into the cells. But this only creates more insulin resistance, in what then becomes a vicious cycle. When the insulin levels can no longer keep pace with rising resistance, blood glucose spikes. That's when your doctor is likely to diagnose type 2 diabetes.

Your doctor may prescribe a medication such as insulin injections, or perhaps a drug called metformin, to lower blood glucose, but *these drugs do not rid the body of excess glucose*. Instead, they simply continue to take the glucose out of the blood and ram it back into the body. It then gets shipped out to other organs, such as the kidneys, the nerves, the eyes, and the heart, where it can eventually create other problems. The underlying problem, of course, is unchanged.

Remember the bowl that was overflowing with sugar? It still is. Insulin has simply moved the glucose from the blood, where you could see it, into the body, where you cannot. So the very next time you eat, sugar spills out into the blood again and you inject insulin to cram it into your body. Whether you think of it as an overstuffed suitcase or an overflowing bowl, it's the same phenomenon all over again.

The more glucose you force your body to accept, the more insulin your body needs to overcome the resistance to it. But this insulin only creates more resistance as the cells become more and more distended. Once you've exceeded what your body can produce naturally, medications can take over. At first, you need only a single medication, but eventually it becomes two and then three, and the doses become larger. And here's the thing: if you are taking more and more medications to keep your blood glucose at the same level, your diabetes is actually getting worse.

Conventional diabetes treatments: How to make the problems worse

The blood glucose got better with insulin, but the diabetes got worse. The medications only hid the blood glucose by cramming it into the already engorged cells. The diabetes *looks* better but actually it is worse.

Doctors may congratulate themselves on the illusion of a job well done, even as patients get sicker. No amount of medication prevents the heart attacks, congestive heart failure, strokes, kidney failure, amputations, and blindness that result when diabetes is getting worse. "Oh well," the doctor says, "it's a chronic, progressive disease."

Here's an analogy. Consider that hiding garbage under your bed instead of discarding it allows you to pretend that your house is clean. When there's no more room under the bed, you can throw the garbage into the closet. In fact, you can hide it anywhere you can't see it: in the basement, in the attic, even in the bathroom. But if you keep hiding your garbage, eventually it's going to begin to smell really, really bad because it's starting to rot. Instead of hiding it, *you need to throw it out.*

If the solution to your overflowing suitcase and your overflowing house seems obvious, the solution to too much glucose, which leads to too much insulin, should also seem self-evident: *Get rid of it!* But the standard treatment for type 2 diabetes follows the same flawed logic of hiding the glucose instead of eliminating it. If we understand that too much glucose in the blood is toxic, why can't we understand that too much glucose in the body is also toxic?

FACT: TYPE 2 DIABETES AFFECTS EVERY ORGAN IN THE BODY

WHAT HAPPENS WHEN excessive glucose piles up in the body over ten or twenty years? Every cell in the body starts to rot, which is precisely why type 2 diabetes, unlike virtually any other disease, affects every single organ. Your eyes rot, and you go blind. Your kidneys rot, and you need dialysis. Your heart rots, and you get heart attacks and heart failure. Your brain rots, and you get Alzheimer's disease. Your liver rots, and you get fatty liver disease and cirrhosis. Your legs rot, and you get diabetic foot ulcers. Your nerves rot, and you get diabetic neuropathy. No part of your body is spared.

Standard medications do not prevent the progression of organ failure because they do not help excrete the toxic sugar load. No less than seven multinational, multicenter, randomized, placebo-controlled trials have proved that standard medications that lower blood glucose do not reduce heart disease, the major killer of diabetic patients. We have pretended that these glucose-lowering medications make people healthier, but it's been a lie. We have overlooked a singular truth: *you can't use drugs to cure a dietary disease.*

FACT: TYPE 2 DIABETES IS REVERSIBLE AND
PREVENTABLE WITHOUT MEDICATIONS

ONCE WE UNDERSTAND that type 2 diabetes is simply too much sugar in the body, the solution becomes obvious. Get rid of the sugar. Don't hide it away. Get rid of it. There are really only two ways to accomplish this.

1. Put less sugar in.
2. Burn off remaining sugar.

That's it. That's all we need to do. The best part? It's all natural and completely free. No drugs. No surgery. No cost.

Step 1: Put less sugar in

The first step is to eliminate all sugar and refined carbohydrates from your diet. Added sugars have no nutritional value and you can safely withhold them. Complex carbohydrates, which are simply long chains of sugars, and highly refined carbohydrates, such as flour, are quickly digested into glucose. The optimum strategy is to limit or eliminate breads and pastas made from white flour, as well as white rice and potatoes.

You should maintain a moderate, not high, intake of protein. When it is digested, dietary protein, such as meat, breaks down into amino acids. Adequate protein is required for good health, but excess amino acids cannot be stored in the body and so the liver converts them into glucose. Therefore, eating too much protein adds sugar to the body. So you should avoid highly processed, concentrated protein sources such as protein shakes, protein bars, and protein powders.

What about dietary fat? Natural fats, such as those found in avocados, nuts, and olive oil—major components of the Mediterranean diet—have a minimal effect on blood glucose or insulin and are well known to have healthy effects on both heart disease and diabetes. Eggs and butter are also excellent sources of natural fats. Dietary cholesterol, which is often associated with these foods, has been shown to have no harmful effect on the human body. Eating dietary fat does not lead to type 2 diabetes or heart disease. In fact, it is beneficial because it helps you feel full without adding sugar to the body.

To put less sugar into your body, stick to whole, natural, unprocessed foods. Eat a diet low in refined carbohydrates, moderate in protein, and high in natural fats.

Step 2: Burn off remaining sugar

Exercise—both resistance and aerobic training—can have a beneficial effect on type 2 diabetes, but it is far less powerful at reversing the disease than dietary interventions. And fasting is the simplest and surest method to force your body to burn sugar.

Fasting is merely the flip side of eating: if you are not eating, you are fasting. When you eat, your body stores food energy; when you fast, your body burns food energy. And glucose is the most easily accessible source of food energy. Therefore, if you lengthen your periods of fasting, you can burn off the stored sugar.

While it may sound severe, fasting is literally the oldest dietary therapy known and has been practiced throughout human history without problems. If you are taking prescription medications, you should seek the advice of a physician. But the bottom line is this:

If you don't eat, will your blood glucose come down? Of course.

If you don't eat, will you lose weight? Of course.

So, what's the problem? None that I can see.

To burn off sugar, a popular strategy is to fast for 24 hours, two to three times per week. Another popular approach is to fast for 16 hours, five to six times per week.

The secret to reversing type 2 diabetes now lies within our grasp. All it requires is having an open mind to accept a new paradigm and the courage to challenge conventional wisdom. You know the basics and are ready to get started. But to really understand why type 2 diabetes is an epidemic and what you can do to effectively manage your own health, read on. Good luck.

PART
ONE

The Epidemic

HOW TYPE 2 DIABETES BECAME AN EPIDEMIC

....

THE WORLD HEALTH Organization released its first global report on diabetes in 2016 and the news was not good. Diabetes was an unrelenting disaster. Since 1980 — a single generation — the number of people around the world afflicted with diabetes has quadrupled. How did this ancient disease suddenly become the twenty-first-century plague?

A SHORT HISTORY OF DIABETES

THE DISEASE OF diabetes mellitus (DM) has been recognized for thousands of years. The ancient Egyptian medical text, *Ebers Papyrus*, written around 1550 BC, first described this condition of "passing too much urine."[1] Around the same time, ancient Hindu writings discussed the disease of *madhumeha*, which loosely translated means "honey urine."[2] Afflicted patients, often children, were mysteriously, inexorably losing weight. Attempts to stop the wasting were unsuccessful despite continual feeding, and the disease was almost uniformly fatal. Curiously, ants were attracted to the urine, which was inexplicably sweet.

By 250 BC, the Greek physician Apollonius of Memphis had termed the condition *diabetes*, which by itself connotes only excessive urination. Thomas Willis added the term *mellitus*, meaning "from honey" in 1675. This descriptor distinguishes diabetes mellitus from a different, uncommon disease known as diabetes insipidus. Most commonly caused by traumatic brain injury, diabetes insipidus is also characterized by excessive urination, but the urine is not sweet. Fittingly, *insipidus* means "bland."

Colloquially, the non-specific term diabetes refers to diabetes mellitus since it is far, far more common than diabetes insipidus. In this book, the term diabetes only refers to diabetes mellitus, and there will be no further discussion of diabetes insipidus.

In the first century AD, the Greek physician Aretaeus of Cappadocia wrote the classic description of type 1 diabetes as a "melting down of flesh and limbs into urine." This summary captures the essential feature of this disease in its untreated form: excessive urine production is accompanied by almost complete wasting away of all tissues. Patients cannot gain weight no matter what they eat. Aretaeus further commented that "life (with diabetes) is short, disgusting and painful" as there was no effective treatment. Once affected, patients followed a predestined, fatal course.

Tasting the urine of the stricken patient for sweetness was the classic diagnostic test for diabetes (ewww...). In 1776, the English physician Matthew Dobson (1732–1784) identified sugar as the substance causing this characteristic sweet taste. The sweetness was found not only in the urine, but also in the blood. Slowly, an understanding of diabetes was unfolding, but a solution was still out of reach.

In 1797, the Scottish military surgeon John Rollo became the first physician to formulate a treatment that carried any reasonable expectation of success. He had observed substantial improvement in a diabetic patient eating an all-meat diet. Given the uniformly grim prognosis of diabetes, this approach was a breakthrough. This extremely low carbohydrate diet was the first diabetic treatment of its kind.

By contrast, French physician Pierre Piorry (1794–1879) advised diabetics to eat large quantities of sugar to replace what they lost in their urine. While the logic seemed reasonable at the time, it was not a successful strategy. A diabetic colleague unfortunate enough to follow this advice later died, and history now only laughs at the good Dr. Piorry.[3] However, this outcome foretold the grim shades of our own highly ineffective advice to follow a high-carbohydrate diet in the treatment of type 2 diabetes.

Apollinaire Bouchardat (1806–1886), who is sometimes called the founder of modern diabetology, established his own therapeutic diet based on the observation that periodic starvation during the Franco-Prussian War of 1870 reduced urinary glucose. His book, *De la Glycosurie ou diabète sucré (Glycosuria or Diabetes Mellitus)* laid out his comprehensive dietary strategy, which forbade all foods high in sugars and starches.

In 1889, Dr. Josef von Mering and Oskar Minkowski at the University of Strasbourg experimentally removed a dog's pancreas, the comma-shaped organ between the stomach and intestine. The dog began to urinate frequently, which Dr. von Mering astutely recognized as a symptom of underlying diabetes. Testing the urine confirmed the high sugar content.

In 1910, Sir Edward Sharpey-Schafer, sometimes regarded as the founder of endocrinology (the study of hormones), proposed that the deficiency of a single hormone he called insulin was responsible for diabetes. The word insulin came from the Latin *insula*, which means "island," as this hormone is produced in cells called the islets of Langerhans in the pancreas.

By the turn of the twentieth century, prominent American physicians Frederick Madison Allen (1879–1964) and Elliott Joslin (1869–1962) became strong proponents of intensive dietary management for diabetes, given the lack of other useful treatments.

Dr. Allen envisioned diabetes as a disease in which the overstrained pancreas could no longer keep up with the demands of an excessive diet.[4] To give the pancreas a rest, he prescribed the "Allen starvation treatment," which was very low in calories (1000 calories per day) and very restricted in carbohydrates (<10g per day). Patients were admitted to hospital and given only whiskey and black coffee every two hours from 7 a.m. to 7 p.m. This regime continued daily until the sugar disappeared from the urine. Why was whiskey included? It was not essential, but was administered simply because it "keeps the patient comfortable while he is being starved."[5]

The response of some patients was unlike anything seen previously. They improved instantly and almost miraculously. Others, however, starved to death, which was euphemistically called inanition.

A lack of understanding of the difference between type 1 and type 2 diabetes severely hampered the usefulness of Allen's treatment. Type 1 diabetic patients were usually dramatically underweight children, whereas type 2 diabetic patients were mostly overweight adults. This ultra-low calorie diet could be deadly for the very malnourished type 1 diabetic (more on the differences between these two types of diabetes below and in chapter 2). Given the otherwise fatal prognosis of untreated type 1 diabetes, this was not the tragedy it may at first have appeared to be. Allen's detractors pejoratively called his treatments starvation diets, but they were widely considered the best therapy, dietary or otherwise, until the discovery of insulin in 1921.

Dr. Elliott P. Joslin opened his practice in 1898 in Boston after receiving his medical degree from Harvard Medical School, becoming the first American doctor to specialize in diabetes. Harvard University's eponymous Joslin Diabetes Center is still considered one of the foremost diabetes institutes in the world, and the textbook Joslin wrote, *The Treatment of Diabetes Mellitus*, is considered the bible of diabetes care. Joslin himself is likely the most famous diabetologist in history.

6   Although Dr. Joslin had lost many patients to diabetes, he had also saved many by applying Dr. Allen's treatments. In 1916, he wrote: "That temporary periods of under-nutrition are helpful in the treatment of diabetes will probably be acknowledged by all after these two years of

experience with fasting."[6] He felt the improvements were so obvious to everybody involved that studies would not even be necessary to prove the point.

THE DISCOVERY OF THE CENTURY

FREDERICK BANTING, CHARLES Best, and John Macleod made the breakthrough discovery of insulin at the University of Toronto in 1921. They isolated insulin from the pancreases of cows and, with James Collip, found a way to purify it enough to administer it to the first patient in 1922.[7] Leonard Thompson, a fourteen-year-old boy with type 1 diabetes, weighed only sixty-five pounds when he started insulin injections. His symptoms and signs rapidly disappeared and he immediately regained a normal weight. They quickly treated six more patients with equally stunning success. The average lifespan of a ten-year-old at diagnosis increased from about sixteen months[8] to thirty-five years!

Eli Lilly and Company partnered with the University of Toronto to commercially develop this revolutionary new drug, insulin. The patent was made freely available so the entire world could benefit from the medical discovery of the century. By 1923, 25,000 patients were being treated with injected insulin, and Banting and Macleod received the Nobel Prize for Physiology or Medicine.

Euphoria ensued. With the momentous discovery of insulin, it was widely believed diabetes had finally been cured. British biochemist Frederick Sanger determined the molecular structure of human insulin, which garnered him the 1958 Nobel Prize in Chemistry and paved the way for the biosynthesis and commercial production of this hormone. Insulin's discovery overshadowed the dietary treatments of the previous century, essentially throwing them into general disrepute. Unfortunately, the story of diabetes did not end there.

It soon became clear that different types of diabetes mellitus existed. In 1936, Sir Harold Percival Himsworth (1905–1993) categorized diabetics based on their insulin sensitivity.[9] He'd noted that some

7

patients were exquisitely sensitive to the effects of insulin, but others were not. Giving insulin to the insulin-insensitive group did not produce the expected effect: instead of lowering blood glucose efficiently, the insulin seemed to have little effect. By 1948, Joslin speculated that many people had undiagnosed diabetes due to insulin resistance.[10]

By 1959, the two different types of diabetes were formally recognized: type 1, or insulin-dependent diabetes, and type 2, or non-insulin dependent diabetes. These terms were not entirely accurate, as many type 2 patients are also prescribed insulin. By 2003, the terms insulin-dependent and non-insulin dependent were abandoned, leaving only the names type 1 and type 2 diabetes.

The names juvenile diabetes and adult-onset diabetes have also been applied, to emphasize the distinction in the age of patients when the disease typically begins. However, as type 1 is increasingly prevalent in adults and type 2 is increasingly prevalent in children, these classifications have also been abandoned.

THE ROOTS OF THE EPIDEMIC

IN THE 1950S, seemingly healthy Americans were developing heart attacks with growing regularity. All great stories need a villain, and dietary fat was soon cast into that role. Dietary fat was falsely believed to increase blood cholesterol levels, leading to heart disease. Physicians advocated lower-fat diets, and the demonization of dietary fat began in earnest. The problem, though we didn't see it at the time, was that restricting dietary fats meant increasing dietary carbohydrates, as both create a feeling of satiety (fullness). In the developed world, these carbohydrates tended to be highly refined.

By 1968, the United States government had formed a committee to look into the issue of hunger and malnutrition across the country and recommend solutions to these problems. A report released in 1977, called *Dietary Goals for the United States,* led to the 1980 *Dietary Guidelines for Americans.* These guidelines included several specific dietary goals, such as raising carbohydrate consumption to 55–60 percent of the diet and decreasing fat consumption from approximately 40 percent of calories to 30 percent.

Although the low-fat diet was originally proposed to reduce the risk of heart disease and stroke, recent evidence refutes the link between cardiovascular disease and total dietary fat. Many high-fat foods, such as avocados, nuts, and olive oil, contain mono- and polyunsaturated fats that are now believed to be heart-healthy. (The most recent *Dietary Guidelines for Americans* released in 2016 have removed restrictions on total dietary fat in a healthy diet.[11])

Similarly, the link between natural, saturated fat and heart disease has been proven false.[12] While artificially saturated fats, such as trans fats, are universally accepted as toxic, the same does not hold true for naturally occurring fats found in meat and dairy products, such as butter, cream, and cheese—foods that have been part of the human diet for time beyond memory.

As it turns out, the consequences of this newfangled, unproven, low-fat, high-carbohydrate diet were unintended: the rate of obesity soon turned upwards and has never looked back.

The 1980 *Dietary Guidelines* spawned the infamous food pyramid in all its counterfactual glory. Without any scientific evidence, the formerly "fattening" carbohydrate was reborn as a healthy whole grain. The foods that formed the base of the pyramid—*foods we were told to eat every single day*—included breads, pastas, and potatoes. These were the precise foods we had previously avoided in order to stay thin. They are also the precise foods that provoke the greatest rise in blood glucose and insulin.

Figure 1.1. Obesity trends in the U.S. after introduction of the "food pyramid"[13]

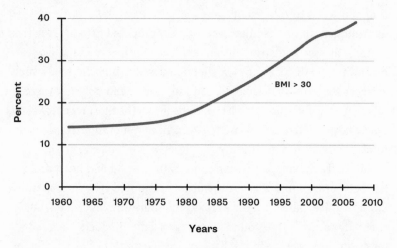

As Figure 1.1 shows, obesity increased immediately. Ten years later, as Figure 1.2 shows, diabetes began its inevitable rise. Age-adjusted prevalence is still rising precipitously. In 1980, an estimated 108 million people worldwide suffered with diabetes. By 2014, that number had swelled to 422 million.[14] Even more concerning is the fact that there seems to be no end in sight.

THE TWENTY-FIRST-CENTURY PLAGUE

DIABETES HAS INCREASED significantly in both sexes, every age group, every racial and ethnic group, and all education levels. Type 2 diabetes attacks younger and younger patients. Pediatric clinics, once the sole domain of type 1 diabetes, are now overrun with an epidemic of obese adolescents with type 2 diabetes.[15]

This is not merely a North American epidemic, but a worldwide phenomenon, although close to 80 percent of the world's adult diabetics live in developing nations.[17] Rates of diabetes are rising fastest in the low- and middle-income nations of the world. In Japan, 80 percent of all new cases of diabetes are type 2.

Figure 1.2. The rising tide of diabetes in the United States[16]

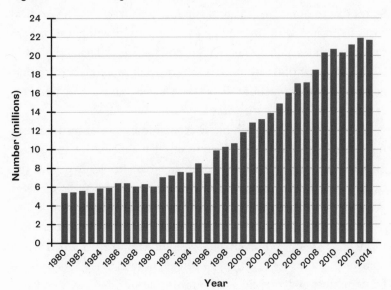

China, in particular, is a diabetes catastrophe. In 2013, an estimated 11.6 percent of Chinese adults had type 2 diabetes, eclipsing even the long-time champion, the U.S., at 11.3 percent.[18] Since 2007, 22 million Chinese—a number close to the population of Australia—have been newly diagnosed with diabetes. This number is even more shocking when you consider that only 1 percent of Chinese had type 2 diabetes in 1980. In a single generation, the diabetes rate has risen by a horrifying 1160 percent. The International Diabetes Federation estimates that the worldwide rate of diabetes will reach 1 in every 10 adults by the year 2040.[19]

The problem is not trivial. In the U.S., 14.3 percent of adults have type 2 diabetes and 38 percent of the population has prediabetes, totaling 52.3 percent. This means that, for the first time in history, more people have the disease than not. Prediabetes and diabetes is the new normal. Worse, the prevalence of type 2 diabetes has increased only in the last forty years, making it clear that this is not some genetic disease or part of the normal aging process but a lifestyle issue.

11

It is estimated that, in 2012, diabetes cost $245 billion in the United States due to direct health costs and lost productivity.[20] The medical costs associated with treating diabetes and all its complications are two to five times higher than treating nondiabetics. Already, the World Health Organization estimates that 15 percent of annual health budgets worldwide are spent on diabetes-related diseases. Those numbers threaten to bankrupt entire nations.

The combination of prohibitive economic and social costs, increasing prevalence, and younger age of onset make obesity and type 2 diabetes the defining epidemics of this century. Ironically, despite the explosion of medical knowledge and technological advances, diabetes poses an even bigger problem today than it did in 1816.[21]

In the 1800s, type 1 diabetes predominated. While almost uniformly fatal, it was relatively rare. Fast-forward to 2016, when type 1 diabetes accounts for less than 10 percent of total cases. Type 2 diabetes dominates and its incidence is growing despite its already endemic nature. Almost all type 2 diabetes patients are overweight or obese and will suffer complications related to their diabetes. Although insulin and other modern medicines can treat blood glucose efficiently, lowering blood glucose alone does not prevent the complications of diabetes, including heart disease, stroke, and cancer—leading causes of death.

That we should have a worldwide epidemic of one of the world's oldest diseases is a bombshell. Whereas all other diseases, from smallpox to influenza to tuberculosis to AIDS, have been controlled over time, the diseases associated with diabetes are increasing at an alarming rate.

But the question still remains: *Why?* Why are we powerless to stop the spread of type 2 diabetes? Why are we powerless to stop the spread among our children? Why are we powerless to stop the ravages of type 2 diabetes on our bodies? Why are we powerless to prevent the heart attacks, strokes, blindness, kidney disease, and amputations that accompany it? More than 3000 years after its discovery, why is there no cure?

The answer is that we have fundamentally misunderstood the disease called type 2 diabetes. To design rational treatments that have a chance of success, we must begin again. We must understand the root causes of the disease, or in medical terms, the aetiology. What is the aetiology of type 2 diabetes? Once we understand that, we can begin. Let us begin.

2

THE DIFFERENCES
BETWEEN TYPE 1 AND
TYPE 2 DIABETES

....

D IABETES MELLITUS COMPRISES a group of metabolic disorders characterized by chronically elevated blood glucose, or hyper-glycemia. The prefix *hyper* means "excessive," and the suffix *emia* means "in the blood," so this term literally means "excessive glucose in the blood."

There are four broad categories of diabetes mellitus: type 1, type 2, gestational diabetes (high blood glucose associated with pregnancy), and other specific types.[1] Type 2 diabetes is by far the most common, making up an estimated 90 percent of cases. Gestational diabetes, by definition, is not a chronic disease, though it increases the future risk of developing type 2 diabetes. If hyperglycemia persists after pregnancy, it must be reclassified as type 1, type 2, or another specific type. Other specific types of diabetes, listed in Table 2.1, are rare. We will not dis-cuss these types of diabetes or gestational diabetes any further in this book.

Table 2.1 Classifications of diabetes mellitus

Type 1
Type 2
Gestational
Other specific types:
- Genetic defects
- Pancreatic disease
- Drug or chemical induced
- Infections
- Endocrinopathies

DIABETES SYMPTOMS

HYPERGLYCEMIA, OR HIGH blood glucose, characterizes all forms of diabetes. When blood glucose levels rise above the kidney's ability to reabsorb the glucose (the renal threshold), it spills over into the urine, causing frequent, excessive urination and severe thirst. The chronic loss of glucose may lead to rapid weight loss and also stimulate the appetite. The most typical symptoms seen in diabetes therefore include

- increased thirst,
- frequent urination,
- rapid, unexplained weight loss,
- increased hunger despite weight loss, and
- fatigue.

These symptoms of hyperglycemia are common to all forms of diabetes, but they occur more frequently in type 1 diabetes, since the onset of type 2 diabetes is typically very gradual. Today, type 2 diabetes is most often diagnosed during routine blood testing, before patients have symptoms.

In severe cases, patients—typically those with type 1 diabetes—may present with diabetic ketoacidosis. Dangerously high levels of acid build up in the blood due to the severe lack of insulin. Symptoms include confusion, rapid breathing, abdominal pain, a fruity smell to one's breath, and loss of consciousness. This is a true emergency situation, which needs immediate treatment with insulin.

Severe cases of type 2 diabetes may present with hyperosmolar non-ketotic syndrome. High blood glucose stimulates excessive urination, leading to severe dehydration, seizures, coma, and even death. Since insulin levels are normal or high in type 2 diabetes, ketoacidosis does not develop.

DIAGNOSING DIABETES

DIABETES MAY BE diagnosed by one of two blood tests: the hemoglobin A1C (often abbreviated to A1C) or the blood glucose. The A1C, which has been accepted as a diagnostic criterion by the American Diabetes Association since 2009, is the most convenient screening test for diabetes because it does not require fasting and can therefore be done at any time of the day.

Hemoglobin A1C

Hemoglobin is a protein found inside red blood cells that carries oxygen to the entire body. Over the average three-month lifespan of a red blood cell, glucose molecules attach to the hemoglobin in proportion to the prevailing blood glucose levels. The amount of glucose attached to the hemoglobin can be measured with a simple blood test called the hemoglobin A1C. The A1C thus reflects the body's average level of blood glucose over three months.

In North America, the A1C is given as a percentage, while in the U.K. and Australia, the units are expressed as mmol/mol. The American Diabetes Association defines an A1C level of 5.7 percent or less to be normal. A level above 6.5 percent is considered diabetic (see Table 2.2).

Table 2.2. Classification of diabetes and prediabetes according to A1C blood glucose levels

A1C	Classification
< 5.7%	Normal
5.7%–6.4%	Prediabetes
> 6.5%	Diabetes

Prediabetes is the in-between stage, where blood glucose levels are abnormally high, but not quite high enough to be considered diabetic. It denotes a state of very high risk of future progression to full-fledged type 2 diabetes. A patient with a baseline A1C of 6.0–6.5 percent (42–48 mmol/mol) has an estimated 25–50 percent risk of developing diabetes within five years. That's more than twenty times the risk of a person with an A1C of 5.0 percent (31 mmol/mol).[2]

Blood glucose

The second test to diagnose diabetes is the blood glucose test, which is also known as the blood sugar or plasma glucose test. It is measured using either a fasting blood sugar test or an oral glucose tolerance test (OGTT).

For the fasting blood glucose test, a patient is asked to have no caloric intake for at least eight hours. A blood sample is then taken and the amount of glucose in the blood is measured. A level above 7.0 mmol/L (or 126 mg/dL) is considered diabetic.

For the OGTT, a patient is asked to ingest a standard test dose of 75 grams of glucose. A blood sample is taken two hours later and the amount of glucose in the blood is measured. A level above 11.1 mmol/L (or 200 mg/dL) is considered diabetic.

17

The A1C has largely replaced the fasting blood glucose test and the OGTT for diagnosis because of its simplicity and convenience, but all of these tests are considered accurate and acceptable. Occasionally, diabetes is diagnosed using a random blood sugar test. A blood sample is taken at a random time and the level of glucose in the blood is measured. A level above 11.1 mmol/L (or 200 mg/dL) is considered diabetic if accompanied by other symptoms.

Table 2.3 Diagnostic criteria for diabetes

Fasting blood glucose > 7.0 mmol/L (126 mg/dL)
2 hour blood glucose > 11.1 mmol/L (200 mg/dL) during OGTT
A1C > 6.5% (48 mmol/mol)
Symptoms of hyperglycemia and random blood glucose > 11.1 mmol/L (200 mg/dL)

The total amount of glucose circulating in the blood at any time is surprisingly small—roughly a single teaspoonful. Glucose does not float freely around in the blood. Rather, most of the body's glucose is contained within our cells.

Hormones tightly regulate our blood glucose to avoid excessively low or high levels. Even when we eat large amounts of sugar, the blood glucose level still remains within a remarkably narrow, controlled range due to the coordinated actions of various hormones. As glucose is absorbed through the intestines into the blood, the islet cells within the pancreas secrete the hormone insulin. Insulin allows the glucose to enter the cells as fuel for energy. The body stores any excess glucose in the liver for future use, which keeps our blood glucose from rising out of its normal range.

TYPE 1 DIABETES: THE FACTS

TYPE 1 DIABETES has been previously called juvenile diabetes, since its onset commonly occurs during childhood. However, although three-quarters of all cases are diagnosed in patients under eighteen, it may present at any age. The global incidence of type 1 diabetes has been rising in recent decades for unknown reasons and may be increasing by as much as 5.3 percent annually in the United States.[3] In Europe, at present rates, new cases of type 1 diabetes will double between 2005 and 2030.

Type 1 diabetes is an autoimmune disease, meaning that the body's own immune system damages the cells that secrete insulin. The patient's blood contains antibodies to normal human islet cells, which provides evidence of an autoimmune attack. Over time, cumulative destruction of the insulin-producing cells causes type 1 diabetes to progress to severe insulin deficiency, whereupon symptoms typically occur.[4]

There is a strong genetic predisposition to type 1 diabetes, but what eventually triggers the autoimmune destruction is uncertain. Seasonal variation in diagnosis may point to an infectious trigger, but which specific one is unclear. Other environmental agents that may play a role include sensitivity to cow's milk, wheat protein, and low vitamin D. Type 1 diabetes often occurs together with other autoimmune diseases, such as Graves' disease (which affects the thyroid) or vitiligo (which affects the skin).

Type 1 diabetics suffer from a severe lack of insulin. Therefore the cornerstone of successful treatment is adequate replacement of the missing hormone insulin. The discovery of insulin injections dramatically improved the prognosis, leading to a widespread feeling that diabetes had been cured. However, the story did not end happily ever after. Over the long term, type 1 diabetics are at much higher risk of complications, which affect almost all organs of the body, than nondiabetics. Type 1 diabetes reduces life expectancy by five to eight years and carries more than ten times the risk of heart disease compared with healthy patients.[5]

TYPE 2 DIABETES: THE FACTS

TYPE 2 DIABETES has historically afflicted older adults, but the prevalence is rising quickly in children worldwide,[6] mirroring the increase in childhood obesity.[7] One clinic in New York City reported a tenfold increase in new cases of diabetes from 1990 to 2000, with half of all new cases being type 2.[8] In 2001, less than 3 percent of newly diagnosed diabetes in adolescents was type 2. Only a decade later, by 2011, this had increased to 45 percent.[9] That is a truly stunning epidemic. In less time than it takes to age a good cheese, type 2 diabetes had risen like a cyclone, leaving only devastation in its wake.

Overall, type 2 diabetes accounts for approximately 90–95 percent of diabetes cases worldwide. It typically develops gradually over many years and progresses in an orderly manner from normal to prediabetes to full-blown type 2 diabetes. The risk increases with age and obesity.

Hyperglycemia occurs due to insulin resistance, rather than the lack of insulin, as in type 1 diabetes. When researchers first developed insulin assays, they expected type 2 diabetes patients to show very low levels, but to their surprise, insulin levels were high, not low.

The failure of insulin to lower blood glucose is called insulin resistance. The body overcomes this resistance by increasing insulin secretion to maintain normal blood glucose levels. The price to be paid is high insulin levels. However, this compensation has a limit. When insulin secretion fails to keep pace with increasing resistance, blood glucose rises, leading to a diagnosis of type 2 diabetes.

DIFFERENT CAUSES REQUIRE DIFFERENT CURES

FUNDAMENTALLY, TYPE 1 and type 2 diabetes are polar opposites, one characterized by very low insulin levels and the other by very high ones. Yet, curiously, standard drug treatment paradigms for the two types are identical. Both primarily target blood glucose, with the goal of lowering it by increasing insulin, even though the high level of blood glucose is only the symptom of the disease and not the disease itself. Insulin helps type 1 diabetes because that disease's underlying core problem is a lack of naturally occurring insulin in the body. However, the underlying core problem of type 2 diabetes is insulin resistance and it remains virtually untreated because there is no clear consensus upon its cause. Without this understanding, we don't have a hope of reversing it. That is our challenge. It may appear formidable, but its rewards are equally enticing: a cure for type 2 diabetes.

3

THE WHOLE
BODY EFFECT

....

D IABETES, UNLIKE VIRTUALLY every other known disease, has
the unique and malignant potential to devastate our entire
body. Practically no organ system remains unaffected by diabetes. These complications are generally classified as either microvascular
(small blood vessels) or macrovascular (large blood vessels).

Certain organs, such as the eyes, kidneys, and nerves, are mostly
supplied by small blood vessels. Damage to these small blood vessels
results in the visual problems, chronic kidney disease, and nerve damage typically seen in patients with long-standing diabetes. Collectively,
these are called microvascular diseases.

Other organs, such as the heart, brain, and legs, are perfused by
large blood vessels. Damage to larger blood vessels results in narrowing
called atherosclerotic plaque. When this plaque ruptures, it triggers the
inflammation and blood clots that cause heart attacks, strokes, and gangrene of the legs. Together, these are known as macrovascular diseases.

How diabetes causes this damage to blood vessels will be discussed
throughout this book. It was widely considered to be simply a consequence of high blood glucose, but the truth, as we'll see, is far different.

Beyond the vascular diseases are many other complications, including skin conditions, fatty liver disease, infections, polycystic ovarian syndrome, Alzheimer's disease, and cancer. However, let's begin with the problems associated with small blood vessels.

MICROVASCULAR COMPLICATIONS

Retinopathy

Diabetes is the leading cause of blindness in the United States.[1] Eye disease—characteristically retinal damage (retinopathy)—is one of the most frequent complications of diabetes. The retina is the light-sensitive nerve layer at the back of the eye that sends its "picture" to the brain. Diabetes weakens the small, retinal blood vessels, which causes blood and other fluids to leak out. During routine physical eye examinations, this leakage can be visualized with a standard ophthalmoscope.

In response to this damage, new retinal blood vessels form, but they are fragile and easily broken. The result is more bleeding and the eventual formation of scar tissue. In severe cases, this scar tissue can lift the retina and pull it away from its normal position, ultimately leading to blindness. Laser treatment can prevent retinopathy by sealing or destroying the leaky new blood vessels.

Approximately 10,000 new cases of blindness in the United States are caused by diabetic retinopathy each year.[2] Whether retinopathy develops depends on how long a person has had diabetes as well as how severe the disease is.[3] In type 1 diabetes, most patients develop some degree of retinopathy within twenty years. In type 2 diabetes, retinopathy may actually develop up to seven years *before* the diabetes itself is diagnosed.

23

Nephropathy

The main job of the kidneys is to clean the blood. When they fail, toxins build up in the body, which leads to loss of appetite, weight loss, and persistent nausea and vomiting. If the disease goes untreated, it eventually leads to coma and death. In the United States, more than 100,000 patients are diagnosed with chronic kidney disease annually, costing $32 billion in 2005. The burden is not only financially enormous, but emotionally devastating.

Diabetic kidney disease (nephropathy) is the leading cause of end stage renal disease (ESRD) in the United States, accounting for 44 percent of all new cases in 2005.[4] Patients whose kidneys have lost over 90 percent of their intrinsic function require dialysis to artificially remove the accumulated toxins in the blood. This procedure involves removing the patient's "dirty" blood, running it through the dialysis machine to clean out its impurities, and then returning the clean blood to the body. To stay alive, patients require four hours of dialysis, three times per week, indefinitely, unless they receive a transplant.

Figure 3.1. Adjusted prevalence rates of end stage renal disease[5]

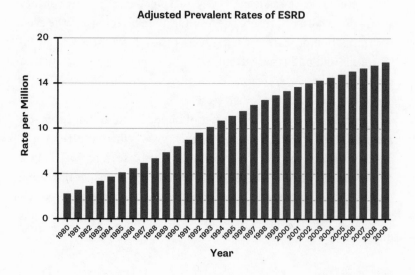

Diabetic kidney disease often takes fifteen to twenty-five years to develop, but, like retinopathy, it may occasionally be diagnosed before type 2 diabetes, itself. Approximately 2 percent of type 2 diabetic patients develop kidney disease each year. Ten years after diagnosis, 25 percent of patients will have evidence of kidney disease.[6] Once established, diabetic nephropathy tends to progress, leading to more and more kidney impairment until eventually the patient requires dialysis or transplantation.

Neuropathy

Diabetic nerve damage (neuropathy) affects approximately 60–70 percent of patients with diabetes.[7] Once again, the longer the duration and severity of diabetes, the greater the risk of neuropathy.[8]

There are many different types of diabetic nerve damage. Commonly, diabetic neuropathy affects the peripheral nerves, first in the feet, and then progressively in the hands and arms as well, in a characteristic stocking-and-glove distribution. Damage to different types of nerves will result in different symptoms, including

· tingling,
· numbness,
· burning, and
· pain.

The incessant pain of severe diabetic neuropathy is debilitating, and the symptoms are commonly worse at night. Even powerful pain-killers such as narcotic medications are often ineffective. Instead of pain, patients may sometimes experience complete numbness. Careful physical examination reveals decreased sensations of touch, vibration, and temperature, and a loss of reflexes in the affected parts of the body.

While a loss of sensation may seem innocuous, it is anything but. Pain protects us against damaging trauma. When we stub our toes, or lie in the wrong position, pain lets us know that we should quickly adjust ourselves in order to prevent further tissue damage. If we are unable to feel pain, we may continue to experience repeated episodes of trauma. Over years, the damage becomes progressive and sometimes deformative. A typical example is the foot. Significant nerve damage

25

can lead to the complete destruction of the joint—a condition called Charcot foot—and may progress to the point where patients are unable to walk, and may even require amputation.

Another nerve disorder affecting the large muscle groups is called diabetic amyotrophy, which is characterized by severe pain and muscle weakness, particularly in the thighs.[9]

The autonomic nervous system controls our automatic body functions, such as breathing, digestion, sweating, and heart rate. Damage to these nerves may cause nausea, vomiting, constipation, diarrhea, bladder dysfunction, erectile dysfunction, and orthostatic hypotension (a sudden, severe drop of blood pressure on standing up). If the nerves to the heart are affected, the risk of silent heart attacks and death increases.[10]

No current treatment reverses diabetic nerve damage. Drugs may help the symptoms of the disease but do not change its natural history. Ultimately, it can only be prevented.

MACROVASCULAR COMPLICATIONS

Atherosclerosis (hardening of the arteries)

Atherosclerosis is a disease of the arteries whereby plaques of fatty material are deposited within the inner walls of the blood vessel, causing narrowing and hardening. This condition causes heart attacks, strokes, and peripheral vascular disease, which are collectively known as cardiovascular diseases. Diabetes greatly increases the risk of developing atherosclerosis.

Atherosclerosis is popularly but incorrectly imagined as cholesterol slowly clogging the arteries, much as sludge might build up in a pipe. In actuality, it results from injury to the artery, although the exact cause of the injury is unknown. There are many contributing factors, including but not limited to age, genetics, smoking, diabetes, stress, high blood pressure, and lack of physical activity. Any breach of the artery's walls can initiate an inflammatory cascade. Cholesterol (a

26

waxy, fat-like substance found in all cells of the body) infiltrates the damaged area and narrows the blood vessel. The smooth muscle that supports the tissue of the blood vessel proliferates, and collagen, a structural protein found abundantly in the body, also accumulates in response to this injury. Again, the result is a further narrowing of the blood vessel. Rather than a single episode that can be simply repaired, this response occurs in reaction to chronic injuries to the vessel wall.

The end result is the development of plaque, known as the atheroma, which is a pocket of cholesterol, smooth muscle cells, and inflammatory cells inside the blood vessel wall. This progressively limits the flow of blood to affected organs. If this atheroma ruptures, a blood clot forms. The sudden blockage of the artery by the clot prevents normal blood circulation and starves the downstream cells of oxygen, causing cell death and cardiovascular disease.

Heart disease

Heart attacks, known medically as myocardial infarctions, are the most well-recognized and feared complication of diabetes. They are caused by atherosclerosis of the blood vessels supplying the heart. The sudden blockage of these arteries starves the heart of oxygen, resulting in the death of part of the heart muscle.

The Framingham studies of the 1970s established a strong association between heart disease and diabetes.[11] Diabetes increases the risk of cardiovascular disease two- to fourfold, and these complications develop at a younger age compared to nondiabetics. Sixty-eight percent of diabetics aged sixty-five or older will die of heart disease, and a further 16 percent will die of stroke.[12] Reducing the risk of macrovascular disease is therefore of primary importance. The extent of death and disability resulting from cardiovascular diseases is many times greater than that resulting from microvascular diseases.

Over the past three decades, there have been significant improvements in the treatment of heart disease, but gains for diabetic patients have lagged far behind. While the overall death rate for nondiabetic men has decreased by 36.4 percent, it has only decreased 13.1 percent for diabetic men.[13]

Stroke

A stroke is caused by atherosclerosis of the large blood vessels supplying the brain. A sudden disruption of the normal blood flow starves the brain of oxygen and a portion of the brain may die. Symptoms vary depending upon which part of the brain is affected, but the devastating impact of stroke cannot be underestimated. In the United States, it is the third leading cause of death and the biggest contributor to disability.

Diabetes is a strong independent risk factor in stroke, meaning that, on its own, diabetes increases a person's risk of having a stroke by as much as 150–400 percent.[14] Approximately a quarter of all new strokes occur in diabetic patients.[15] Every year of diabetes increases the risk of stroke by 3 percent,[16] and the prognosis is also far worse.

Peripheral vascular disease

Peripheral vascular disease (PVD) is caused by atherosclerosis of the large blood vessels supplying the legs. The disruption of normal blood flow starves the legs of oxygen-carrying hemoglobin. The most common symptom of PVD is pain or cramping that appears with walking and is relieved by rest. As the blood vessels narrow and circulation worsens, pain may also appear at rest and especially at night. PVD significantly reduces mobility, which can lead to long-term disability.

Skin with a poor blood supply is more likely to be damaged and takes longer to heal. In diabetics, minor cuts or injuries to the feet may become non-healing foot ulcers. In severe cases, these areas where the skin has broken down, revealing underlying tissue, can progress to gangrene. At this point, blood supply has been greatly reduced or completely lost, the tissue dies, and amputation of the affected limb—a treatment of last resort—often becomes necessary to treat chronic infections and relieve pain.

Diabetes, along with smoking, is the strongest risk factor for PVD. Approximately 27 percent of diabetic patients with PVD will progressively worsen over a five-year period, and 4 percent of them will need an amputation.[17] Patients with gangrene and those requiring amputation may never walk again, which can result in a cycle of disability. A loss of function of the limbs leads to less physical activity, which in turn leads to progressive deconditioning of the muscles. Weaker muscles lead to less physical activity, and the cycle repeats.

OTHER COMPLICATIONS

Alzheimer's disease

Alzheimer's disease is a chronic, progressive, neurodegenerative disease that causes memory loss, personality changes, and cognitive problems. It is the most common form of dementia, and the sixth leading cause of death in the United States.[18] Alzheimer's disease may reflect the inability to use glucose normally, perhaps a type of selective insulin resistance in the brain. The links between Alzheimer's disease and diabetes have grown so strong that many researchers have suggested Alzheimer's disease can be called type 3 diabetes.[19] These arguments go far beyond the scope of this book, however.

Cancer

Type 2 diabetes increases the risk of most common cancers, including breast, stomach, colorectal, kidney, and endometrial cancers. This may be related to some of the medications used to treat diabetes and will be further discussed in chapter 10. The survival rate of cancer patients with pre-existing diabetes is far worse than for nondiabetics.[20]

Fatty liver disease

Non-alcoholic fatty liver disease (NAFLD) is defined as the storage and accumulation of excess fat in the form of triglycerides exceeding 5 percent of the total weight of the liver. This condition can be detected

29

using an ultrasound to examine the abdomen. When this excess fat causes damage to the liver tissue, which can be revealed through standard blood tests, it is called non-alcoholic steatohepatitis (NASH). Current estimates suggest that NAFLD affects 30 percent and NASH 5 percent of the U.S. population; both are important causes of liver cirrhosis (irreversible scarring of the liver).[21]

NAFLD is virtually non-existent in recent-onset type 1 diabetes. By contrast, the incidence in type 2 diabetes is estimated at upwards of 75 percent. The central role of fatty liver is more fully explained in chapter 7.

Infections

Diabetics are more prone to all types of infections, which are caused by foreign organisms invading and multiplying in the body. Not only are they more susceptible to many types of bacterial and fungal infections than nondiabetics, the effects also tend to be more serious. For example, diabetics have a four- to fivefold higher risk of developing a serious kidney infection.[22] All types of fungal infections, including thrush, vaginal yeast infections, fungal infections of the nails, and athlete's foot, are more common in diabetic patients.

Among the most serious infections for diabetics are those involving the feet. Despite adequate blood glucose control, 15 percent of all diabetic patients will develop non-healing foot wounds during their lifetime. Infections in these wounds often involve multiple microorganisms, making broad-spectrum antibiotic treatment necessary. However, the decreased blood circulation associated with PVD (see above) contributes to the poor wound healing. As a result, diabetics have a fifteen-fold increased risk of lower-limb amputation, and account for over 50 percent of the amputations done in the United States, excluding accidents. It is estimated that each of these cases of infected diabetic foot ulcers costs upwards of $25,000 to treat.[23]

There are many contributing factors to the higher rates of infection. High blood glucose may impair the immune system. As well, poor blood circulation decreases the ability of infection-fighting white blood cells to reach all parts of the body.

Skin and nail conditions

Numerous skin and nail conditions are linked to diabetes. Generally, they are more of an aesthetic concern than a medical one; however, they often indicate the underlying serious condition of diabetes, which requires medical management.

Acanthosis nigricans is a gray-black, velvety thickening of the skin, particularly around the neck and in body folds, caused by high insulin levels. Diabetic dermopathy, also called shin spots, are often found on the lower extremities as dark, finely scaled lesions. Skin tags are soft protrusions of skin often found on the eyelids, neck, and armpits. Over 25 percent of patients with skin tags have diabetes.[24]

Nail problems are also common in diabetic patients, particularly fungal infections. The nails may become yellowy-brown, thicken, and separate from the nail bed (onycholysis).

Erectile dysfunction

Community-based population studies of males aged 39–70 years found that the prevalence of impotence ranges between 10 and 50 percent. Diabetes is a key risk factor, increasing the risk of erectile dysfunction more than threefold and afflicting patients at a younger age than usual. Poor blood circulation in diabetics is the likely reason for this increased risk. The risk of erectile dysfunction also increases with age and severity of insulin resistance, with an estimated 50–60 percent of diabetic men above the age of 50 having this problem.[25]

Polycystic ovarian syndrome

An imbalance of the hormones can cause some women to develop cysts (benign masses) on the ovaries. This condition, called polycystic ovarian syndrome (PCOS), is characterized by irregular menstrual cycles, evidence of excessive testosterone, and the presence of cysts (usually

31

detected by ultrasound). PCOS patients share many of the same characteristics as type 2 diabetics, including obesity, high blood pressure, high
cholesterol, and insulin resistance. PCOS is caused by elevated insulin
resistance[26] and increases the risk of developing type 2 diabetes three-
to fivefold in young women.

TREAT THE CAUSE, NOT THE SYMPTOMS

WHEREAS MOST DISEASES are limited to a single organ system, diabetes affects every organ in multiple ways. As a result, it is the leading
cause of blindness. It is the leading cause of kidney failure. It is the
leading cause of heart disease. It is the leading cause of stroke. It is the
leading cause of amputations. It is the leading cause of dementia. It is
the leading cause of infertility. It is the leading cause of nerve damage.

But the perplexing question is why these problems are getting *worse*,
not better, even centuries after the disease was first described. As our
understanding of diabetes increases, we expect that complications
should decrease. But they don't. If the situation is getting worse, then
the only logical explanation is that our understanding and treatment
of type 2 diabetes is fundamentally flawed.

We focus obsessively on lowering blood glucose. But high blood
glucose is only the symptom, not the cause. The root cause of the
hyperglycemia in type 2 diabetes is high insulin resistance. Until we
address that root cause, insulin resistance, the epidemic of type 2 diabetes and all of its associated complications will continue to get worse.

We need to start again. What causes type 2 diabetes? What causes
insulin resistance and how can we reverse it? Obviously, obesity plays
a large role. We must begin with the aetiology of obesity.

SIMON

....

When he came to the Intensive Dietary Management (IDM)
program, Simon, 66, weighed 267 pounds, with a waist circumference of 135 cm and a BMI of 43. He had been diagnosed with
type 2 diabetes eight years earlier and was taking the medications
sitagliptin, metformin, and glicizide to control his blood glucose. In
addition, he had a history of high blood pressure and part of one
kidney had been removed because of cancer.

We counseled him on a low-carbohydrate, healthy-fat diet and
suggested that he start fasting for 24 hours, three times per
week. Within six months, he was down to a single medication,
canagliflozin, which he continued taking for a period of time to help
with weight loss. After another year, we discontinued this medication as Simon's weight and blood glucose had significantly
improved. He has not needed any medications since.

At his last checkup, Simon's hemoglobin A1C was 5.9%, which
is considered nondiabetic, and he had maintained a 45-pound
weight loss for two years and counting. Today, he is ecstatic about
the change in his overall health. He has gone from wearing a size
46 pant to a 40, and the type 2 diabetes, which he believed was a
lifelong disease, has completely reversed. Simon continues to follow a low-carbohydrate diet and fasts once or twice per week for
24 hours.

BRIDGET

When we first met Bridget, 62, she had a ten-year history of type 2 diabetes, chronic kidney disease, and high blood pressure. She was severely insulin resistant, requiring a total of 210 units of insulin every day to keep her blood glucose under control. She weighed 325 pounds, with a waist size of 147 cm and a BMI of 54.1.

Determined to get off insulin, she started with a seven-day fast but felt so well and so empowered that she continued for another two weeks. By the end of the 21 days, she had not only stopped all her insulin but required no diabetic medications at all. To maintain her weight loss, she switched from fasting continuously to fasting for 24 to 36 hours every other day, and she resumed taking dapagliflozin to help control her weight. During this time her A1C was 6.8%, which was actually better than when she was taking insulin.

Before starting the IDM program, Bridget had very low energy levels and could barely make it into my office on her own two legs. Once she started to fast, her energy levels improved significantly and she was easily able to walk around. Her dress size dropped from size 30 to 22. Bridget has been off insulin for three years now and has maintained a total weight loss of 63 pounds over that time. Her blood pressure has normalized and she has stopped taking medication.

(PART TWO)

Hyperinsulinemia
and Insulin Resistance

4

DIABESITY: THE CALORIE DECEPTION

....

IABESITY IS THE unification of the words diabetes, referring to type 2, and obesity. Just like the evocative "bromance," it conveys the close relationship between these two ideas. Diabetes and obesity are truly one and the same disease. As strange as it may now sound, physicians did not always recognize this seemingly obvious and basic connection.

Back in 1990, when grunge was taking over the music scene and fanny packs were growing in popularity beyond the middle-aged dad tourist, Dr. Walter Willett, now Professor of Epidemiology and Nutrition at Harvard's School of Public Health, identified the strong and consistent relationship between weight gain and type 2 diabetes.

The obesity epidemic had only just gotten underway in the late 1970s and was not yet the public health disaster it is today. Type 2 diabetes barely scratched the surface as a public health concern. Instead, AIDS was the hot topic of the day. And type 2 diabetes and obesity were not thought to be related in any way. Indeed, the *Report of the Dietary Guidelines Advisory Committee* issued by the U.S. Department of Agriculture in 1990 allowed that some weight gain after the age of thirty-five was consistent with good health.

That same year, Dr. Willett challenged the conventional thinking, reporting that weight gain after age eighteen was the major determinant of type 2 diabetes.[1] A weight gain of 20–35 kg (44–77 pounds) increased the risk of type 2 diabetes by 11,300 percent. Gaining more than 35 kg (77 pounds) increased the risk by 17,300 percent! Even smaller amounts of weight gain could raise the risk significantly. But this idea was not an easy sell to a sceptical medical profession.[2] "We had a hard time getting the first paper published showing that even slight overweight greatly increased the risk of diabetes," Willett remembers. "They didn't believe it."

BODY MASS INDEX: THE RELATIONSHIP
BETWEEN OBESITY AND DIABETES

THE BODY MASS index is a standardized measurement of weight, and it is calculated by the following formula:

Body mass index = Weight (kg)/Height^2 (m^2)

A body mass index of 25.0 or higher is considered overweight, while a body mass index of between 18.5 and 24.9 is in the healthy range.

Table 4.1. Body mass index classifications

Body Mass Index	Classification
< 18.5	Underweight
18.5–24.9	Normal weight
25.0–29.9	Overweight
30.0–34.9	Obese
35.0–39.9	Severe Obesity
> 40.0	Morbid Obesity

However, women with a body mass index of 23–23.9 have a 360-percent higher risk of developing type 2 diabetes than women with a body mass index of less than 22, which is even more stunning since a body mass index of 23.9 is considered well within the normal weight range.

By 1995, building on this new realization, researchers had determined that a weight gain of only 5.0–7.9 kg (11–17.5 pounds) increased the risk of type 2 diabetes by 90 percent, and a weight gain of 8.0–10.9 kg (17.5–24 pounds) increased the risk by 270 percent.[3] By contrast, weight loss decreased risk by more than 50 percent. This result established an intimate relationship between weight gain and type 2 diabetes. But far more sinister, this excess weight also significantly increased the risk of death.[4]

More supporting evidence would soon surface. Dr. Frank Speizer from the Harvard School of Public Health had established the original Nurses' Health Study (NHS) in 1976. One of the largest investigations into risk factors for cardiovascular disease and cancer, this long-term epidemiological study included 121,700 female nurses from around the Boston area.

Dr. Willett continued with the Nurses' Health Study II, which collected data every two years on an additional 116,000 female nurses since 1989. At the start of the study, all the participants were relatively healthy, but over time, many of them developed chronic diseases such as diabetes and heart disease. By looking back at the collected data, some idea of the risk factors for these diseases emerged. In 2001, Dr. Willett[5] showed that, once again, the single most important risk factor for the development of type 2 diabetes was obesity.

GLYCEMIC INDEX: DIET AND DIABETES

THE NURSES' HEALTH Study II revealed that other lifestyle variables were also important. Maintaining a normal weight, getting regular physical exercise, not smoking, and eating a healthy diet could prevent a stunning *91 percent* of type 2 diabetes. But the million-dollar question is: *What is a "healthy" diet?* Dr. Willett's healthy diet was defined as high in cereal fiber, high in polyunsaturated fats, low in trans fat, and low in glycemic load.

When digested, carbohydrates break down into glucose. The glycemic index measures the rise in blood glucose after ingesting 50 grams of carbohydrate-containing foods. However, the amount of carbohydrates contained in a standard serving varies enormously. For example, a standard serving of fruit may contain less than 50 grams of carbohydrates whereas a single pastry may contain far more. The glycemic load refines this measure by multiplying the glycemic index of a food by the grams of carbohydrate in a standard serving of that food.

Generally, foods high in sugar and refined carbohydrates are high in glycemic load. Dietary fats and proteins, since they raise blood glucose very little, have minimal glycemic loads. Contrary to the low-fat diet recommended by all the medical associations around the world, Dr. Willett's healthy diet was *high* in dietary fat and protein. His diet was about reducing *sugar and refined carbohydrates*, not reducing dietary fat.

In 1990, the widespread belief was that dietary fat was evil, that dietary fat was a mass murderer, that dietary fat was vile. The term healthy fats did not exist. It was an oxymoron, like a jumbo shrimp. Fat-laden avocados? A heart attack in a fruit. Fat-laden nuts? A heart attack in a snack. Olive oil? Liquid heart attacks. Most people fervently believed fats were going to clog our arteries, but it was only an illusion.

Dr. Zoë Harcombe, a Cambridge University–trained obesity researcher, reviewed all the data that had been available in the early 1980s, when low-fat guidelines were introduced in the U.S. and U.K. No proof had *ever* existed that natural dietary fats worsened cardiovascular disease. The evidence for the low-fat guidelines was simply a great work of fiction.[6] The science was far from settled at the time the government decided to weigh in and make the final decision to vilify dietary fat. Yet this belief had become so entrenched both in the medical establishment and among the general public that it had become heretical to suggest refined grains and sugars were the problem rather than dietary fat.

40

In the midst of our frenzied low-fat obsession, Dr. Willett's asser-
tion was considered high treason. But the truth could not be concealed
forever. Today, we understand clearly that obesity is the main underlying issue behind type 2 diabetes. But the problem isn't simply obesity.
Rather, it is *abdominal* obesity.

WAIST CIRCUMFERENCE: FAT DISTRIBUTION
AND TYPE 2 DIABETES

IN 2012, DR. Michael Mosley was a TOFI. A what? Not tofu, the delicious Asian soy delicacy. The acronym TOFI stands for "thin on the
outside, fat on the inside." Dr. Mosley is a medical doctor, British Broad-
casting Corporation (BBC) journalist, documentary filmmaker, and
international bestselling author. And, in his mid-50s, he was also a
ticking time bomb.

He was not particularly overweight, weighing 187 pounds, standing 5 feet 11 inches, with a waist of 36 inches. This equals a body mass
index of 26.1, just barely in the overweight range. By standard measurements, he was considered just fine. He felt fine, perhaps carrying a little
bit of weight around the mid-section from being middle-aged. Just a
little pudge, that's all.

However, body mass index is not the best indicator of type 2 diabetes risk. The waist circumference, a measure of body fat distribution
around the trunk, is a far superior predictor of type 2 diabetes.[7] Filming
a health segment for the BBC, Mosley underwent a magnetic resonance
imaging (MRI) body scan. To his shock and consternation, his organs
were literally swimming in fat. To look at him, you would not have
guessed it because most of the fat was hidden inside his abdomen.

Eighteen months later, during a visit to his own physician, routine
screening blood tests revealed type 2 diabetes. Devastated, Dr. Mosley
says, "I had assumed I was healthy and suddenly I was discovering I
wasn't, and had to take this visceral fat situation seriously."[8] Visceral
fat accumulates inside and around the intra-abdominal organs such as
the liver, kidneys, and intestines, and can be detected by an increased

waist circumference. This pattern of obesity, where most of the fat is carried around the abdomen, is also known as central obesity, or central adiposity. In contrast, subcutaneous fat is the fat deposited directly under the skin.

The different health risks associated with the different fat distributions explain how roughly 30 percent of obese adults are metabolically normal.[9] These healthy-fat people carry more subcutaneous fat rather than the more dangerous visceral fat. On the other hand, some normal-weight people show the same metabolic abnormalities as in obesity[10] because of excessive visceral fat.

Type 2 diabetes may be diagnosed for patients with a wide range of body mass indexes, following a normal distribution with no distinct subpopulation of "thin" diabetics.[11] A full 36 percent of newly diagnosed diabetics have a normal body mass index of less than 25. Look at Figure 4.1. The key clinical indicator is clearly not total body fat as measured by body mass index. Rather, it's visceral or intra-organic fat.[12]

Figure 4.1. Population BMI distribution for newly diagnosed diabetes[13]

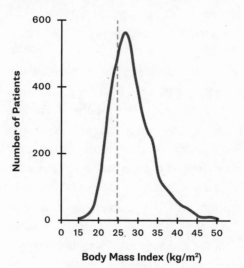

Independent of total weight, central obesity is highly correlated to metabolic abnormalities,[14] increased cardiac risk,[15] and progression to type 2 diabetes.[16] Reducing visceral fat also successfully reduces the risk of progression of type 2 diabetes.[17]

Subcutaneous fat, on the other hand, shows little correlation to type 2 diabetes or heart disease. The surgical removal, via liposuction,[18] of almost 10 kilograms of subcutaneous fat brought no significant metabolic benefits whatsoever, which suggests that subcutaneous fat plays little role in the development of type 2 diabetes.

The waist-to-height ratio is a simple measure of central adiposity, calculated by comparing waist circumference to height. This ratio is far more predictive of years of life lost than body mass index.[19] Optimally, your waist circumference should be less than half your height. For example, an average man standing 5 foot 10 inches (70 inches) should strive to maintain a waist size of 35 inches or less. As central obesity increases, risk of metabolic disease skyrockets.

Figure 4.2. Waist-to-height ratio and years of life lost (YLL): A dramatic increase[20]

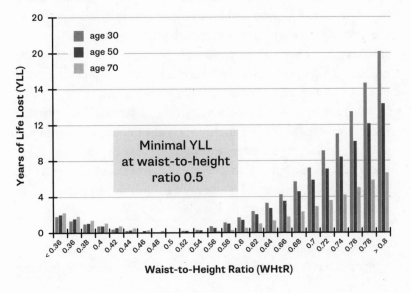

43

There is a distinction even between types of visceral fat. Fat found inside the organs, such as within the liver and pancreas, is called intra-organic fat and is distinctly more dangerous than fat found around the organs, called omental fat. Intra-organic fat increases the risk for the metabolic complications of obesity, including type 2 diabetes, NASH (non-alcoholic steatohepatitis, or fatty liver disease), and cardiovascular disease.[21] On the other hand, surgical removal of omental fat does not result in any metabolic improvement.[22]

Fat within the liver, called intrahepatic fat, plays a crucial role in the development of insulin resistance.[23] Central obesity tracks very closely with intrahepatic fat content.[24] Fat within the pancreas also plays a leading role in type 2 diabetes, as we will see in chapter 7.

So, given the principal role of central obesity, what drives this fat deposition into the organs? Isn't it all about calories?

CALORIE CONFUSION: NO RELATIONSHIP BETWEEN DIABETES AND CALORIES

EAT LESS. CUT your calories. Watch your portion size. These mantras have formed the foundation of conventional weight-loss advice over the past fifty years. And the widespread obesity epidemic proves that this advice has been an utter disaster, perhaps only topped by the nuclear meltdown of Chernobyl. This caloric reduction advice is based on a false understanding of what causes weight gain.

What causes obesity? We don't stop to consider this basic question because we believe that we already know the full answer. It seems so obvious, doesn't it? Excessive intake of calories causes obesity. Too many calories in compared to too few calories out leads to weight gain. This energy balance model of obesity has been drilled into us since childhood.

Fat Gained = Calories In − Calories Out

For the past fifty years, our best weight-loss advice was primarily to restrict our caloric intake. Specifically, we were told to restrict the amount of dietary fat, which is calorically dense. This means reducing foods high in fat, such as meat, butter, cheese, and nuts, in order to lower our calorie intake and therefore lose weight. We made food guides, food pyramids, and food plates to indoctrinate children into this brand-new, low-calorie religion. "Cut Your Calories," we declared. "Eat Less, Move More," we chanted.

Nutrition labels were mandated to include calorie counts. Programs and apps were created to more precisely count calories. We invented small devices such as Fitbits to measure exactly how many calories we were burning. Using all our ingenuity, focused like a laser beam and dogged as a turtle crossing a road, we cut calories.

What was the result? Did the problem of obesity simply fade away like the morning mist on a hot summer day? In a word, no. The underlying, unspoken premise of this model is that energy creation (calories in), energy expenditure (calories out), and fat gain are independent variables fully under our conscious control. It assumes that the number of calories used to keep our bodies running more or less normally remains stable and unchanging. But this is untrue.

The truth is that the body can adjust its basal metabolic rate (BMR)—the energy required to keep the heart pumping, lungs breathing, kidneys and liver detoxifying, brain thinking, body generating heat, and so on—up or down by 40 percent. When you eat fewer calories, your body slows down so it uses fewer calories, *which means you don't lose weight.*

This model also completely ignores the multiple overlapping hormonal systems that signal hunger and satiety. That is, we may decide what to eat and when to eat it, but we cannot decide to *feel* less hungry. We cannot decide when to burn calories as body heat and when to store them as body fat. Hormones make these decisions. The results of the so-called "caloric reduction as primary" advice could hardly have been worse if we had tried. The storm of obesity and type 2 diabetes that began in the late 1970s has today, some forty years later, become a global category 5 hurricane threatening to engulf the entire world in sickness and disability.

Only two possibilities can explain how obesity could spread so rapidly in the face of our shiny new advice to reduce fat and calories: first, perhaps this advice is good but people are simply not following it; second, perhaps the advice is simply wrong.

The idea that the spirit is willing but the flesh is weak—that people have the dream but not the drive—is as absurd as expecting a drowning man to laugh.

Was the entire obesity epidemic simply a sudden, simultaneous, coordinated, worldwide lack of willpower? The world can't agree which side of the road we should drive on, yet, without discussion, we all decided to eat more and move less so that we could become undesirably fat? This explanation is only the latest iteration of the game called "blame the victim." It shifts the responsibility from the advice giver (the advice is bad) to the advice taker (the advice is good, but you are not following it).

By declaring that their scientifically unproven caloric reduction advice was flawless, doctors and nutritionists could conveniently shift the blame from themselves to you. It wasn't *their* fault. It was *yours*. *Their* advice was good. *You* didn't follow it. No wonder they love this game so much. To admit that all their precious theories of obesity were simply incorrect was too psychologically difficult. Yet evidence continued to accumulate that this new caloric restriction strategy was about as useful as a comb to a bald man.

The Women's Health Initiative[25] was the most ambitious, important nutrition study ever done. This randomized trial involving almost 50,000 women evaluated the low-fat, low-calorie approach to weight loss. Although it was not specifically a weight-loss trial, one group of women was encouraged through intensive counseling to reduce their daily caloric intake by 342 calories and to increase their level of exercise by 10 percent. These calorie counters expected a weight loss of 32 pounds every single year.

When the final results were tallied in 1997, there was only crushing disappointment. Despite good compliance, more than seven years of calorie counting had led to virtually no weight loss. Not even a single pound. This study was a stunning and severe rebuke to the caloric theory of obesity. Reducing calories did not lead to weight loss.

There were now two choices. First, we could respect the expensive, hard-won, scientific evidence to devise a robust, more correct theory of obesity. Or we could simply keep all our comfortable and convenient preconceived notions and biases and ignore the science. The second choice involved far less work and far less imagination. So this ground-breaking study has largely been ignored and relegated to the dustbins of nutritional history. We have been paying the pied piper every day since, as the twin epidemics of obesity and type 2 diabetes have exploded.

Real-world studies[26] have only confirmed this stunning fiasco. The conventional weight-loss advice to eat fewer calories carries an estimated failure rate of 99.4 percent. For morbid obesity, the failure rate is 99.9 percent. These statistics would not surprise anybody in the diet industry or, for that matter, anybody who has ever tried to lose weight.

The Calories-In, Calories-Out theory gained widespread acceptance based on its seemingly intuitive truth. However, like a rotting melon, digging past the outer shell revealed the putrid interior. This simplistic formula is riddled with erroneous assumptions. The most important error is believing that basal metabolic rate, or Calories Out, always remains stable. But a 40-percent reduction in calorie intake is quickly met with a 40-percent decrease in basal metabolic rate. The net result is no weight loss.

The other major false assumption is that weight is consciously regulated. But no system in our body functions like that. The thyroid, parathyroid, sympathetic, parasympathetic, respiratory, circulatory, hepatic, renal, gastrointestinal, and adrenal systems are all closely controlled by hormones. Body weight and body fat are also strictly regulated by hormones. In fact, our bodies contain multiple overlapping systems of body weight control. Body fat, one of the most important determinants of survival in the wild, is simply not left to the vagaries of what we decide to put in our mouths.

47

HORMONES: FOOD, BODY WEIGHT, AND DIABETES

HORMONES CONTROL HUNGER, telling our body when to eat and when to stop. Ghrelin is a powerful hormone that causes hunger, and cholecystokinin and peptide YY are hormones that tell us when we are full and should stop eating. Imagine you're at an all-you-can-eat buffet. You've already eaten many heaping platefuls of food and you are completely, 110-percent full.

Now, could you eat a few more pork chops? Merely the thought might make you nauseous. Yet these are the same pork chops you ate happily just a few minutes ago. The difference is that satiety hormones are exerting a powerful effect to stop you from eating. Contrary to many popular beliefs, we do not continue eating simply because food is available. Calorie consumption is under tight hormonal regulation.

Fat accumulation is truly not a problem of energy excess. It's a problem of energy *distribution*. Too much energy is diverted to producing fat as opposed to, say, increasing body heat or forming new bone tissue. This energy expenditure is controlled hormonally. As long as we believed, wrongly, that excessive caloric intake led to obesity, we were doomed to failure as we uselessly tried to reduce calories.

We cannot "decide" to feel less hungry. We cannot "decide" to increase basal metabolic rate. If we eat fewer calories, our body simply compensates by decreasing its metabolic rate. If calories are not the underlying cause of weight gain, then reducing calories cannot reliably reduce weight. The most important factor in controlling fat accumulation and weight gain is to control the hormonal signals we receive from food, not the total number of calories we eat.

Obesity is a hormonal imbalance, not a caloric one. The hormonal problem in undesired weight gain is mainly excessive insulin. Thus, type 2 diabetes, too, is a disease about insulin imbalance rather than caloric imbalance.

5

THE ROLE OF INSULIN IN ENERGY STORAGE

....

ERE'S A STARTLING fact: I can make you fat. Actually, I can make anybody fat. How? It's really quite simple. I prescribe insulin. Although insulin is a natural hormone, excessive insulin causes weight gain and obesity.

Hormones are essentially chemical messengers. They are produced by the endocrine system, a network of glands found throughout the body to maintain proper function. The pea-sized pituitary gland in the brain is often called the master gland because it produces many different hormones that control metabolic processes in other parts of the body. For example, it secretes growth hormone, which signals the rest of the body, including the bones and muscles, to grow bigger. The butterfly-shaped thyroid gland in the neck produces thyroid hormone to deliver its message to the rest of the body. When it receives this signal, the heart may beat faster, breathing may accelerate, and the basal metabolic rate may increase. Similarly, the pancreas produces insulin, a hormone that delivers several different messages mostly relating to the intake and storage of food energy.

INSULIN BASICS

WHEN WE EAT, foods are broken down in the stomach and small intestine for easier absorption. All foods are composed of three main constituents, called macronutrients. These are proteins, fats, and carbohydrates, and they are all handled differently by the digestive system. Proteins are broken down into amino acids. Fats are broken down into fatty acids. Carbohydrates, composed of chains of sugars, are broken down into smaller sugars, including glucose. Micronutrients, as the name implies, are nutrients that are necessary for good health in far smaller quantities, such as vitamins and minerals.

One of insulin's roles is to facilitate the uptake of glucose into cells for energy, by opening a channel to allow it inside. Hormones find their target cell by binding to receptors on the cell surface, much like a key fitting into a lock. Only the correct hormone can open the receptor and deliver the message. Insulin works like the key, fitting snugly into the lock on the cell to open a gateway for glucose. Every cell in the body can use glucose for energy. Without insulin, glucose circulating in the blood cannot easily enter the cell.

In type 1 diabetes, autoimmune destruction of insulin-secreting cells leads to abnormally low levels of insulin. Without keys to open the gates, glucose cannot enter to provide energy for the cell and builds up in the bloodstream, even as the cell faces internal starvation. As a result, patients continually lose weight, no matter how much they eat, since they are unable to properly use the available food energy. Unused, this glucose is eventually excreted in the urine, even as the patient wastes away. Untreated, type 1 diabetes is usually fatal.

When people without type 1 diabetes eat, insulin rises, and glucose enters the cell to help us meet our immediate energy needs. The excess food energy is stored away for later use. Some carbohydrates, particularly sugars and refined grains, raise blood glucose effectively, which stimulates the release of insulin. Dietary protein also raises insulin levels, but not blood glucose, by simultaneously raising other hormones, such as glucagon and incretins. Dietary fats only minimally raise both blood glucose and insulin levels.

Another of insulin's key roles is to signal to the liver that nutrients are on their way. The intestinal bloodstream, known as the portal circulation, delivers amino acids and sugars directly to the liver for processing. On the other hand, fatty acids are absorbed directly and do not pass through the liver before entering into the regular bloodstream. Since liver processing is not required, insulin signaling is not necessary and insulin levels remain relatively unchanged by pure dietary fats.

Once our immediate energy needs have been met, insulin gives the signal to store food energy for later use. Our body uses dietary carbohydrates to provide energy for working muscles and the central nervous system, but the excess also provides glucose to the liver. Amino acids are used to produce protein, such as muscle, skin, and connective tissue, but the liver converts the excess into glucose, since amino acids cannot be stored directly.

Food energy is stored in two forms: glycogen and body fat. Excess glucose, whether derived from protein or from carbohydrates, is strung together in long chains to form the molecule glycogen, which is stored in the liver. It can be converted to and from glucose easily and released into the bloodstream for use by any cell in the body. Skeletal muscles also store their own glycogen, but only the muscle cell storing the glycogen can use it for energy.

The liver can only stockpile a limited amount of glycogen. Once it is full, the excess glucose is turned into fat by a process called de novo lipogenesis (DNL). *De novo* means "from new" and *lipogenesis* means "making new fat," so this term means literally "to make new fat." Insulin triggers the liver to turn excess glucose into new fat in the form of triglyceride molecules. The newly created fat is exported out of the liver to be stored in fat cells to supply the body with energy when it is required. In essence, the body stores excess food energy in the form of sugar (glycogen) or body fat. Insulin is the signal to stop burning sugar and fat and to start storing it instead.

This normal process occurs when we stop eating (and begin fast-ing), which is when the body needs this source of energy. Although we often use the word fasting to describe periods in which we deliberately limit certain foods or abstain from eating altogether, such as before a medical procedure or in conjunction with a religious holiday, it simply applies to any period between snacks or meals when we are not eating. During periods of fasting, our body relies on its stored energy, meaning that it breaks down glycogen and fat.

Figure 5.1. Storage of food energy as sugar or fat

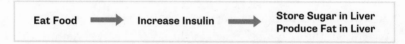

Several hours after a meal, blood glucose drops and insulin lev-els begin to fall. To provide energy, the liver starts to break down the stored glycogen into component glucose molecules and releases it into general circulation in the blood. This is merely the glycogen-storage process in reverse. This happens most nights, assuming you don't eat at night.

Glycogen is easily available but in limited supply. During a short-term fast (twenty-four to thirty-six hours), glycogen will provide all the glucose necessary for normal body functioning. During a pro-longed fast, the liver will manufacture new glucose from stored body fat. This process is called *gluconeogenesis*, meaning literally "the making of new sugar." In essence, fat is burned to release energy. This is merely the fat-storage process in reverse.

Figure 5.2. Gluconeogenesis: The reverse of the glycogen storage process

| Burn Stored Sugar in Liver
Burn Fat in Liver | ← | Decrease Insulin | ← | No Food
"Fasting" |

This energy storage-and-release process happens every day. Normally this well-designed, balanced system keeps itself in check. We eat, insulin goes up, and we store energy as glycogen and fat. We fast, insulin goes down, and we use our stored glycogen and fat. As long as feeding (insulin high) is balanced with fasting (insulin low), no overall fat is gained.

Insulin has another role related to storage. When the liver is full of glycogen, there is no room for the newly created fat from DNL. These triglyceride molecules are packaged together with specialized proteins, called lipoproteins, which are made in the liver and exported into the bloodstream as very low-density lipoprotein (VLDL). Insulin activates the hormone lipoprotein lipase (LPL), which signals offsite fat cells, called adipocytes, to remove the triglycerides from the blood for long-term storage. In this manner, excess carbohydrates and protein can be stored long term offsite as body fat.

Excessive insulin drives fat accumulation and obesity. How? If our feeding periods predominate over our fasting periods, then the ensuing insulin dominance leads to fat accumulation. Too much insulin signals the liver to keep admitting glucose, resulting in more production of new fat via DNL. Normally, if periods of high insulin (feeding) alternate with periods of low insulin (fasting), weight remains stable. If high insulin persists, the body receives the constant signal to store food energy as body fat.

INSULIN: THE CAUSE OF WEIGHT GAIN AND OBESITY

INSULIN IS PRESCRIBED to lower blood glucose in both type 1 and type 2 diabetes. Virtually every patient taking insulin and every prescribing physician knows full well that weight gain is the main side effect. This is strong evidence that hyperinsulinemia, high levels of insulin in the blood, directly causes weight gain. But there is other corroborating evidence as well.

Insulinomas are rare tumors that continually secrete very high levels of insulin. These cause low blood glucose and persistent weight gain, underscoring insulin's influence once again. Surgical removal of these tumors results in weight loss. Similarly, sulfonylureas are diabetic medications that stimulate the body to produce more of its own insulin. With insulin stimulation, weight gain is the main side effect. Although the thiazolidinedione (TZD) drug class, used to treat type 2 diabetes, does not increase insulin levels, it does increase insulin's effect. The result? Lower blood glucose, but also weight gain.

Weight gain, however, is not an inevitable consequence of treating diabetes. Currently, metformin is the most widely prescribed medication worldwide for type 2 diabetes. Rather than increasing insulin, it blocks the liver's production of glucose (gluconeogenesis) and therefore reduces blood glucose. It successfully treats type 2 diabetes without increasing insulin and, therefore, does not lead to weight gain.

Where excessively high insulin levels lead to weight gain, excessively low insulin levels lead to weight loss. Remember, patients with untreated type 1 diabetes have pathologically low insulin levels and no matter how many calories they ingest, they cannot gain any weight. Without normal levels of insulin, these patients cannot properly use or store food energy and, untreated, they waste away and die. With the replacement of insulin, these patients gain weight once again.

Increasing insulin causes weight gain. Decreasing insulin causes weight loss. These are not merely correlations but direct causal factors. Our hormones, mostly insulin, ultimately set our body weight and level of body fat. *Remember, obesity is a hormonal imbalance, not a caloric one.*

THE CARBOHYDRATE-INSULIN HYPOTHESIS

HYPERINSULINEMIA CAUSES OBESITY. This point is crucial because it immediately makes obvious that successful treatment of obesity depends upon lowering insulin levels. Highly refined, processed carbohydrates—sugars, flour, bread, pasta, muffins, donuts, rice, and potatoes—are well known to raise blood glucose and insulin production. If these highly refined carbohydrates were the main cause of hyperinsulinemia, they would also be the prime cause of weight gain. This theory of obesity is known as the carbohydrate-insulin hypothesis. It forms the rational basis for many low-carbohydrate diets, such as the Atkins diet. By eliminating many of the "fattening" carbohydrates, we lower insulin levels and prevent weight gain.

Figure 5.3. Hormonal obesity I: Hyperinsulinemia causes obesity

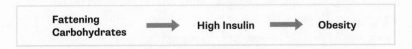

As you read the coming chapters, watch the progression of the "Hormonal Obesity" diagrams from this one through Figures 5.4, 6.3, 7.2, 8.1, 9.1, 9.2, 9.3, and 9.4). Reviewed in sequence, these diagrams illustrate how the building blocks of the metabolic syndrome stack up over time.

The first low-carbohydrate diet dates all the way back to the mid-nineteenth century. In 1863, William Banting (1796–1878), an English undertaker, published the pamphlet *Letter on Corpulence, Addressed to the Public*,[1] which is often considered the world's first diet book. Weighing 202 pounds (91.6 kilograms), Banting had tried unsuccessfully to lose weight by eating less and exercising more. But, just like today's dieters, he was unsuccessful.

On the advice of his surgeon, Banting tried a new approach. When he strenuously avoided the bread, milk, beer, sweets, and potatoes that had previously made up a large portion of his diet, he lost weight and successfully kept it off. For most of the next century, diets low in refined carbohydrates were accepted as the standard treatment for obesity.

For all the success of low-carb diets, the carbohydrate-insulin hypothesis remains incomplete. While refined carbohydrates are certainly an important contributor to hyperinsulinemia, they are not the *only* contributor. There are many other significant influences. One of the most important is insulin resistance.

As we've seen, insulin acts like a key to open a gate for glucose to enter the cell. But sometimes, in a state of insulin resistance, the usual levels of insulin are not sufficient and glucose piles up in the blood-stream because it cannot get into the cells. To compensate, the body produces more insulin to overcome this resistance and force the blood glucose inside. The effect is to restore normal blood glucose levels but at a cost of persistent hyperinsulinemia. We care about insulin resistance so much because this compensatory hyperinsulinemia drives overall weight gain. But here's the million-dollar question: How does this insulin resistance develop in the first place?

Figure 5.4. Hormonal obesity II: Insulin resistance causes hyperinsulinemia

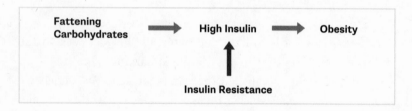

6

INSULIN RESISTANCE: THE OVERFLOW PHENOMENON

....

O BESITY TYPICALLY PRECEDES the diagnosis of type 2 diabetes by a decade or more. Obese but otherwise normal (nondiabetic) patients have substantially increased insulin resistance compared to lean patients. Fasting insulin, a measure of the amount of insulin in the blood that reflects underlying insulin resistance, increases through the spectrum of obesity, prediabetes, and then type 2 diabetes (see Figure 6.1).[1]

This suggests that obesity could be the root cause of increased insulin resistance. But despite spending millions of dollars and doing decades of intensive research on possible hormonal mediators between obesity and insulin resistance, no causal link could be made. After all, if obesity causes insulin resistance, how could type 2 diabetes develop in normal-weight patients? And why do so many obese people *not* develop type 2 diabetes?

Figure 6.1. Changes in insulin as obesity progresses toward type 2 diabetes[2]

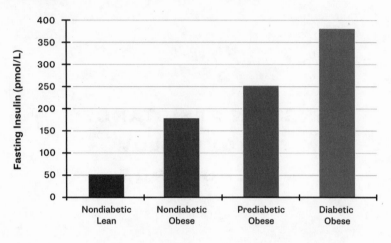

The converse, the idea that insulin resistance causes obesity, is implausible since obesity typically predates insulin resistance. The only remaining possibility is that some X factor is the underlying cause of both obesity and insulin resistance. The connection, as we shall see, is too much insulin. The X factor is hyperinsulinemia.

Figure 6.2. Hyperinsulinemia: The X factor causing both obesity and insulin resistance

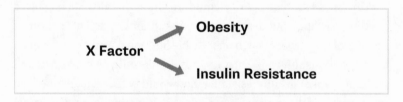

58   **RESISTANCE AS A PROTECTIVE MECHANISM**

THE HUMAN BODY follows the fundamental biological principle of homeostasis. If things change too far in one direction, the body reacts by changing in the opposite direction to try to return to its original state. For instance, if we become very cold, the body adapts by shivering to generate more body heat. If we become very hot, the body sweats to cool itself. Adaptability is a prerequisite for survival and generally holds true for all biological systems.

Resistance is simply another word for this adaptability. The body resists change out of its comfort range by adapting to it. Exposure creates resistance. Excessively high and prolonged levels of anything provoke resistance by the body. This is a normal phenomenon. Consider the following.

Laura was only 25 when she was diagnosed with an insulinoma,[3] a rare tumor that secretes abnormally large amounts of insulin in the absence of any other significant disease. This condition forces glucose into the cells, causing recurrent episodes of hypoglycemia, or low blood glucose. As a result, Laura was constantly hungry and, as insulin is a major driver of obesity, she soon began to gain weight.[4] Her glucose levels were too low to maintain adequate brain function, which led to problems with concentration and coordination. One night, as she was driving, she lost control of her feet and narrowly avoided an accident. She had experienced a seizure related to hypoglycemia.

Laura's symptoms may appear severe, but they would have been much worse if her body had not taken protective steps. As her insulin levels increased, insulin resistance increased in lock step. Without insulin resistance, her high insulin levels would rapidly have led to very, very low blood glucose and death. Since the body doesn't want to die (and neither do we), it protects itself by developing insulin resistance, demonstrating homeostasis. The resistance develops naturally to shield against the unusually high insulin levels. *Insulin causes insulin resistance.* Fortunately, the correct diagnosis was soon made and she had corrective surgery. With the tumor removed, insulin resistance dramatically reverses, as do associated conditions.[5]

Reversing the high insulin levels also reverses insulin resistance. Exposure creates resistance. Removing the stimulus also removes the resistance. This rare disease gives us a vital clue in understanding the cause of insulin resistance.

HOW RESISTANCE WORKS

HOMEOSTASIS IS SO fundamental to survival that the body will find many different ways to develop resistance. Survival depends on it. Let's take a look at a few different resistance mechanisms.

Noise resistance

The very first time you yell at somebody, they jump back and pay attention. Incessant yelling, though, soon negates its effect. In essence, they have developed resistance. The boy who cried wolf soon learned that the villagers became resistant to its effect. *Exposure creates resistance.*

Removing the stimulus removes the resistance. What happens when the yelling stops? If the boy stopped crying wolf for a month, the villagers would start listening again. This prolonged silence reverses the resistance. The next time he cries wolf, it will have an immediate effect.

Have you ever watched a baby sleep in a crowded, noisy airport? The ambient noise is very loud, but constant, and the baby sleeps soundly, as it has become resistant to the noise. That same baby sleeping in a quiet house might awaken at the slightest creak of the floorboards. This is every parent's worst nightmare. Even though it is not loud, the noise is very noticeable, as the baby has no resistance. The baby immediately wakes up crying, to the parents' dismay.

Antibiotic resistance

When new antibiotics are introduced, they eradicate virtually all the bacteria they're designed to kill. Over time, most bacteria develop the ability to survive high doses of these antibiotics, which turns them into drug-resistant "superbugs." As the superbugs multiply and become more prevalent, the antibiotic loses its effectiveness. This is a large and growing problem in many urban hospitals worldwide. Every single antibiotic has lost effectiveness due to resistance.

Antibiotic resistance is not a new phenomenon. Scottish biologist Alexander Fleming discovered penicillin in 1928 and mass production began in 1942, with funds from the U.S. and British governments, for use during World War II. In his 1945 Nobel lecture, "Penicillin," Dr. Fleming correctly predicted the emergence of resistance two years before the first cases were reported.

How did Dr. Fleming so confidently predict this development? He understood the fundamental biological principle of homeostasis. A biological system that becomes disturbed tries to go back to its original state. As we use an antibiotic more and more, organisms resistant to it are naturally selected to survive and reproduce. Eventually, these resistant organisms dominate, and the antibiotic becomes useless. Persistent, high-level use of antibiotics causes antibiotic resistance. *Exposure creates resistance.*

Removing the stimulus removes the resistance. Unfortunately, the knee-jerk reaction of many doctors is just the opposite: to prescribe more antibiotics to overcome the resistance, which backfires and creates even more resistance. Preventing antibiotic resistance means severely restricting their use. This has led many hospitals to develop steward- ship programs to preserve the effect of the most powerful antibiotics by using them *only* in life-threatening situations. Lowering the exposure of bacteria to the antibiotic creates less resistance, which can save lives.

Viral resistance

Resistance to viruses such as diphtheria, measles, chicken pox, or polio develops from the viral infection itself. Before the development of vac- cines, it was popular to hold "measles parties" or "pox parties," where unaffected children would play with a child who was actively infected with the virus in order to deliberately expose them. Not the funnest of parties, but having measles once protects a child for life. *Exposure creates resistance.*

61

Vaccines work on this exact principle. Edward Jenner, a young doctor working in rural England, heard the common tale of milkmaids developing resistance to the fatal smallpox virus because they had contracted the milder cowpox virus. In 1796, he deliberately infected a young boy with cowpox and observed how he was subsequently protected from smallpox, a similar virus. By being inoculated with a dead or weakened virus, we build up immunity without actually causing the full disease. In other words, viruses cause viral resistance.

Drug resistance

When a drug such as cocaine is taken for the first time, there is an intense reaction—the "high." With each subsequent use of the drug, this high becomes progressively less intense. Drug abusers may start to take larger doses to achieve the same high. Through repeated and prolonged exposure, the body develops resistance to the drug's effects, a condition called tolerance. People can build up resistance to many different types of drugs, including narcotics, marijuana, nicotine, caffeine, alcohol, benzodiazepines (tranquilizers), and nitroglycerin. Again, *exposure creates resistance.*

Removing the stimulus removes the resistance. In order to restore sensitivity to the medication, it is necessary to have a period of low drug use. If you stop drinking alcohol for a year, the first drink afterwards will have its full effect again.

What do all of these examples have in common? In the case of noise, stimulus fatigue is the mechanism of resistance. The human ear responds to changes rather than the absolute noise levels. In the case of antibiotics, the natural selection of resistant organisms is the mechanism. The bacteria that adapt to the drugs are the ones that survive and multiply. In the case of viruses, the development of antibodies is the mechanism of resistance. In the case of drug resistance, or desensitization, a decrease in the number of cell receptors is the mechanism. While the mechanism in each of these cases may differ, the end result is always the same. That's the point. Homeostasis is so fundamental to survival that biological systems always find a way to compensate. *Exposure creates resistance.*

And what does this tell us about insulin resistance? *Insulin causes insulin resistance.*

HOW INSULIN CAUSES INSULIN RESISTANCE

HORMONES, SUCH AS insulin, act much like drugs when it comes to resistance. Both act upon cell surface receptors, and they show the same phenomenon of resistance. In the case of insulin, prolonged and excessive exposure to this hormone—hyperinsulinemia—causes insulin resistance. Proving it experimentally is quite simple. Take a group of healthy volunteers, give them persistent, high doses of insulin, and look for resistance to develop. Luckily, all the experiments have already been done.

In one study, a forty-hour constant insulin infusion into a group of healthy young people increased insulin resistance by 15 percent.[6] In a similar experiment, a ninety-six-hour constant intravenous infusion of insulin into a group of healthy young people increased insulin resistance by 20 to 40 percent.[7] The implications of these results are simply staggering. Giving normal but persistent amounts of insulin alone to these healthy young people made them insulin resistant. *Insulin causes insulin resistance.* That is, I can make *anybody* insulin resistant. All I need to do is give them enough insulin.

In type 2 diabetes, giving large doses of insulin produces increased insulin resistance. In one study, patients initially not taking insulin were titrated up to a very high dose of 100 units of insulin per day.[8] The higher the insulin dose, the more insulin resistance they developed—a direct causal relationship, as inseparable as a shadow is from a body. Even as blood glucose levels got better, the diabetes was getting worse. *Insulin causes insulin resistance.*

However, high hormonal levels *by themselves* cannot cause resistance or we would all quickly develop crippling levels of resistance. Our

63

bodies naturally defend against resistance by secreting our hormones in short bursts. High levels of hormones are released at specific times to produce a specific effect. Afterwards, the levels quickly drop and stay very low. This is the body's daily circadian rhythm. The prolonged low periods of hormone ensure that resistance does not develop.

For example, the hormone melatonin, produced by the pineal gland to regulate our sleep and wake cycles, is virtually undetectable during the day. As night falls, it increases to peak in the early morning hours. Cortisol, produced by the adrenal glands to regulate stress, spikes just before we wake up and then drops down to low levels. Growth hormone, produced in the pituitary gland to help us regenerate cells, is secreted mostly in deep sleep and then falls to undetectable levels during the day. Parathyroid hormone, which regulates bone metabolism, peaks in the early morning. The periodic release of these and other hormones is essential in preventing resistance.

Hormone levels generally stay very low. Every so often a brief pulse of the specific hormone, often triggered by the circadian rhythm, comes along to create maximum effect. After it passes, our levels are very low again. The brief pulse of hormone is over long before resistance has a chance to develop. The body does not continuously cry wolf. When it does on occasion, we experience the full effect.

For resistance to develop, two essential factors are required: high hormonal levels and constant stimulus. Normally, insulin is released in bursts, preventing insulin resistance from developing. But when the body is constantly bombarded with insulin, resistance develops.

It should be obvious by now that, since resistance develops in *response* to high, persistent levels of a stimulus, raising the dose only leads to more resistance. It's a vicious, self-reinforcing cycle: *exposure creates resistance.* Resistance leads to higher exposure. Higher exposure increases resistance. When constant high levels of insulin "yell" for glucose to enter the cell, it has progressively less effect (insulin resistance). The body's knee-jerk reaction is to produce even more insulin—to yell even louder. The louder it yells, the less effect it has. Hyperinsulinemia drives the vicious cycle. Hyperinsulinemia leads to insulin resistance, which leads to worsening hyperinsulinemia.

Figure 6.3. Hormonal obesity III: High insulin → resistance → higher insulin

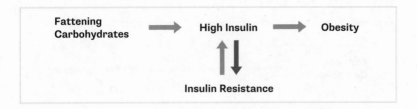

The cycle keeps going around and around, until the insulin levels in the body are extremely high, which drives weight gain and obesity. The longer the cycle continues, the worse it becomes, which is why obesity and insulin resistance are so time dependent. People can be stuck in this vicious cycle for decades, developing significant insulin resistance. Resistance then leads to high insulin levels, which are *independent of diet*.

But the story gets worse. Insulin resistance leads to higher *fasting* insulin levels. Fasting insulin levels are normally low. Now, instead of starting the day with low insulin after the nightly fast, we start with high insulin. The consequences are dire: the fat get fatter. As insulin resistance becomes a larger and larger part of the problem, it can, in fact, become a major driver of high insulin levels. *Obesity drives itself.*

The fact that insulin resistance leads to compensatory hyper-insulinemia has been long accepted. But the novel notion that hyperinsulinemia also causes insulin resistance is slowly gaining acceptance. Dr. Barbara Corkey, the 2011 Banting Medal winner from Boston University's School of Medicine, called her lecture, "Hyperinsu-linemia is the root cause of insulin resistance, obesity and diabetes."[9] The Banting Medal is the American Diabetes Association's highest sci-entific award, so these are not merely the musings of a fringe group.

The hallmark of type 2 diabetes is elevated insulin resistance. Both obesity and type 2 diabetes are manifestations of the same underlying problem: hyperinsulinemia. Their close relationship has given rise to the term "diabesity," which implicitly acknowledges that they are one and the same disease.

Figure 6.4. Hyperinsulinemia: The link between obesity and diabetes

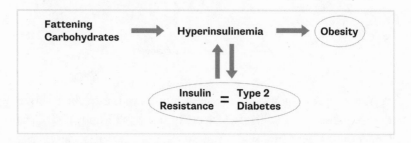

HYPERINSULINEMIA AND THE OVERFLOW PHENOMENON

INSULIN RESISTANCE OCCURS when blood glucose remains elevated despite normal or high levels of insulin, since the cells are resisting insulin's pleas to take up glucose. But how does hyperinsulinemia cause this phenomenon?

The currently held lock-and-key paradigm suggests that the key (insulin) opens the lock (cell surface receptor) to allow glucose inside, and that once you remove the key (insulin), blood glucose can no longer enter the cell. With insulin resistance, we imagine that the lock and key no longer fit together very well. The key only partially opens the lock and not very easily, so glucose, which cannot enter normally, instead piles up outside, in the blood. As less glucose enters the cell, it faces a state of internal starvation and the body produces more insulin. Since each key works less efficiently, the body compensates by producing more keys. This hyperinsulinemia ensures that enough glucose gets into the cells to meet its energy requirement. It's a nice, neat theory. Too bad it has no basis in reality.

66

Is the problem the key (insulin) or the lock (insulin receptor)? Well, neither. The molecular structure of both insulin and the insulin receptor is completely normal in type 2 diabetes. Therefore, something must be gumming up the lock-and-key mechanism. But what? Despite decades of intensive research, no plausible culprit has been positively identified.

Recall that insulin goes up when you eat and acts predominantly in the liver to help store incoming food energy. Insulin instructs the liver to do two things:

1. Stop burning stored food energy (e.g. body fat).
2. Store incoming food energy as glycogen or produce new fat via de novo lipogenesis (DNL).

If the cell were truly resistant to insulin and suffering internal starvation, both actions should be simultaneously blunted. This certainly holds true for the first action of insulin. Insulin yells at the liver to stop making new glucose, but the liver continues to pump it out. Glucose spills out into the blood.

However, the second action of insulin is paradoxically enhanced. If glucose cannot enter the cell, causing internal starvation, then the liver has no substrate to create new fat and DNL should shut down. How can the liver make new fat from glucose if it has no glucose? It's like trying to build a brick house with no bricks. Even if you have construction workers, it is impossible.

With insulin resistance, DNL actually *increases*, so insulin's effect is not blunted but accelerated. So much new fat is being generated that there is nowhere to put it. This excess fat accumulates in the liver, where there normally should be none at all. With insulin resistance, liver fat should be *low*, not high. But type 2 diabetes is almost always associated with excessive fat accumulation in the liver.

How can the liver selectively resist one of insulin's effects yet accelerate the other? And in the very same cell, in response to the very same levels of insulin, with the very same insulin receptor? Despite decades of ongoing research and millions of dollars, all the world's top researchers were still stumped by this central paradox of insulin resistance

67

until they realized that the old gummed-up, lock-and-key paradigm of insulin resistance with internal starvation was incorrect. The vital clue is that insulin itself causes insulin resistance, which means that the primary problem is *not* insulin resistance but the hyperinsulinemia that caused it.

Insulin resistance only refers to the fact that, for a given amount of insulin, it is more difficult to move glucose into the cell. So what if *the glucose cannot enter the cell because it is already overflowing?* The paradigm of insulin resistance as an overflow phenomenon resolves the central paradox.

HOW THE OVERFLOW PHENOMENON WORKS

PICTURE A SUBWAY train at rush hour. The train stops at a station, gets the all-clear signal from the conductor, and opens its doors to let passengers on. All the passengers enter the train without difficulty and the platform is empty as the train pulls away.

The cell is like the subway train, insulin is like the conductor, and the glucose molecules are like the passengers. When insulin gives the proper signal, the gates open and glucose enters the cell in an orderly fashion without much difficulty. With an insulin-resistant cell, insulin signals the cell to open the gate, but no glucose enters. Glucose accumulates in the blood, unable to get inside. What has happened?

Consider our train analogy. The train pulls into the station and receives the signal to open the doors, but no passengers get on. This is "conductor" resistance. As the train pulls away, many passengers are left standing on the platform. Under the lock-and-key paradigm, the conductor's signal fails to open the subway doors fully because something is jamming the mechanism. Passengers can't get through the doors and they are left on the platform while the empty train pulls away.

The overflow phenomenon suggests a different possibility. The train pulls into the station but it is already jam-packed with passengers from the previous stop. When the conductor gives the signal to open the door, the passengers waiting on the platform cannot get on *because the train is already full*. From our view on the outside, we only see that passengers cannot enter the train and conclude that the door did not open.

The same situation occurs in the liver cell. If high insulin levels have already jammed the cell full of glucose, no more can enter even if insulin opens the gate. From the outside, we can only say that the cell is now *resistant* to insulin's urging to move glucose inside.

In our train analogy, one way to pack more people into the train is to hire "subway pushers." In New York City in the 1920s, people were forcibly shoved into the packed trains. While this practice has died out in North America, it still exists in Japan. When passengers are left standing on the platform, "passenger arrangement staff" push more people onto the train.

Hyperinsulinemia is the body's subway pusher. It shoves glucose into the already stuffed cell. When glucose is left outside, the body produces extra insulin to forcibly push more glucose into the cell. This tactic works at first, but as more and more glucose is forced inside

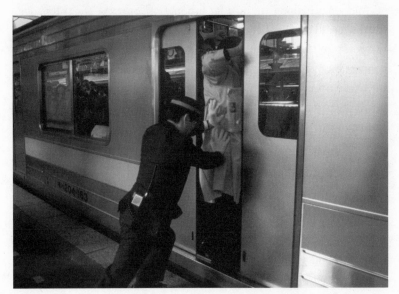

the overstuffed cell, more force is required. Insulin resistance causes compensatory hyperinsulinemia. But what was the initial cause? Hyperinsulinemia. It's a vicious cycle.

Let's think about the liver cell. At the beginning, the cell (train) is empty. If equal amounts of glucose (passengers) enter and leave, then everything works normally. If feeding (insulin high) and fasting (insulin low) periods are balanced, insulin resistance does not develop.

With persistent hyperinsulinemia, glucose (passengers) keeps entering the cell (train) and not leaving. Over time, the cell (train) overflows and glucose (passengers) cannot enter even when the cell surface receptor (door) is open. The cell is now insulin resistant. To compensate, the body produces more insulin (subway pushers) to force more glucose inside, but over time this only makes it worse by creating higher insulin resistance.

Insulin resistance creates hyperinsulinemia, and vice versa. The vicious cycle goes around and around. The cell is not in a state of internal starvation; instead, it is overflowing with glucose. As it spills out of the cell, blood glucose levels increase.

And what happens to new fat production, or DNL? The cell is overfilled with glucose, not empty, so there is no reduction of DNL. Instead, the cell produces as much new fat as possible to relieve the internal congestion of glucose. If more new fat is created than can be exported, fat backs up in the liver, an organ not designed for fat storage. The result is fatty liver. This overflow paradigm perfectly explains the central paradox.

Looking at blood glucose, the cell appears insulin resistant. Looking at DNL, the cell appears to have enhanced insulin sensitivity. This happens in the liver cell, with the same level of insulin and the same insulin receptors. The paradox has been resolved by understanding this new paradigm of insulin resistance. The cell is not internally starved; it is overloaded with glucose. The physical manifestation of that cell—overstuffed with excess glucose, now turned into fat via DNL—can be seen as fatty infiltration of the liver.

70

Figure 6.5. Too much sugar → fatty liver → insulin resistance

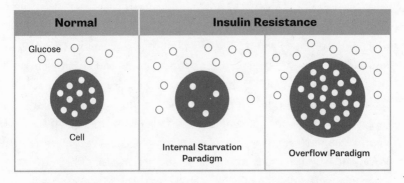

Insulin resistance is predominantly a glucose overflow problem of the overstuffed, fatty liver. As the first stop for metabolism of ingested nutrients, the liver is naturally the epicenter of health problems related to excess consumption. Insulin resistance is primarily caused by excessive fatty infiltration of the liver caused in turn by excessive glucose and fructose consumption. In other words, too much sugar causes fatty liver, the key problem of insulin resistance, as Figure 6.5 shows.

PHILIP

Philip, 46, had been admitted to hospital to receive intravenous antibiotics for a non-healing diabetic foot ulcer. He'd already had the ulcer for ten months and, despite constant dressings and care from the plastic surgeon, it had become infected. At the time, he had a five-year history of type 2 diabetes and was taking sitagliptin and metformin to control his blood glucose. I spoke with Philip and his father in the hospital about the gravity of his situation, since non-healing ulcers often destroy the foot, eventually leading to amputation.

Once Philip completed his antibiotics and was discharged from the hospital, I asked him to attend the IDM program. Fasting is a regular part of the Greek Orthodox religion he practices, and so he quickly understood the logic of our program. He started fasting once a week for 48 hours, and within a month he was able to stop taking both of his blood glucose medications because his readings were normal. His "chronic, non-healing" ulcer healed within a month.

Philip has been following the IDM program for a year, and takes no medications. His ulcers have not recurred, he has lost 20 pounds, and his A1C is only 6.5%, which is below the 7.2% he had achieved even with two medications.

SYBIL

Sibyl, 69, had a ten-year history of type 2 diabetes as well as high blood pressure, heart attack, stroke, and triple bypass surgery. When I met her, she had been taking insulin for five years and required 70 units daily, in addition to sitagliptin and metformin to keep her blood glucose in check. She weighed 202 pounds and had a waist circumference of 117 cm, with a BMI of 35.8.

On the IDM program she started a low-carbohydrate, healthy-fat diet, along with alternating 24- and 36-hour fasts every other day. Her doctor carefully managed her insulin dose to avoid both high and low blood glucose, and closely monitored her overall health. In two months, she was able to stop taking all her insulin and also the sitagliptin. Now, six months into the program, she has lost 30 pounds and 13 cm off her waist. She is still working toward getting off her diabetes medications entirely, but her A1C measures 6.2% and her dose of metformin has been reduced accordingly.

(PART THREE)

Sugar and the
Rise of Type 2 Diabetes

7

DIABETES, A DISEASE
OF DUAL DEFECTS

....

THE ENGLISH FRIAR and philosopher, William of Ockham (1287–1347), is credited with developing the fundamental problem-solving principle known as *lex parsimoniae*, or "Ockham's razor." This postulate holds that the hypothesis with the fewest assumptions is often true. In other words, the simplest explanation is usually correct. Albert Einstein is quoted as saying, "Everything should be made as simple as possible, but not simpler."

While type 2 diabetes is considered primarily a disease of excessive insulin resistance, it actually represents two separate physiological defects. First, insulin resistance, an overflow phenomenon, is caused by fatty infiltration of the liver and muscle. Insulin resistance develops early in the disease process, typically preceding the diagnosis of type 2 diabetes by a decade or more, but blood glucose remains relatively normal because the pancreatic beta cells increase insulin production to balance. This compensatory hyperinsulinemia forces the glucose into the cells, keeping blood glucose levels normal.

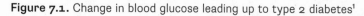

Figure 7.1. Change in blood glucose leading up to type 2 diabetes[1]

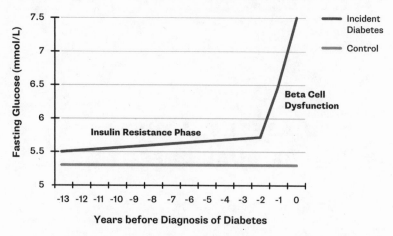

Without dietary intervention, this insulin resistance almost always leads to the second problem, beta cell dysfunction. Furthermore, only insulin resistance and virtually nothing else causes beta cell dysfunction. Conventional medical wisdom holds that this dysfunction occurs because of exhaustion and eventual scarring of the insulin-producing cells. This idea implies that these two phenomena—insulin resistance and beta cell dysfunction—occur for entirely separate reasons. However, given this mutually exclusive and intimate relationship, Ockham's razor suggests that both defects must surely be caused by the same underlying mechanism.

Only when insulin production fails to keep pace with increasing resistance does the blood glucose rise high enough to make the clinical diagnosis of type 2 diabetes. Thus, there are two underlying prerequisites of the disease: elevated insulin resistance *and* beta cell dysfunction. The progression of blood glucose levels in the years preceding the diagnosis occurs in two distinct phases, reflecting these two distinct abnormalities.[2]

PHASE 1: HYPERINSULINEMIA / INSULIN RESISTANCE

AS SHOWN IN Figure 7.1, insulin resistance emerges, on average, almost thirteen years prior to type 2 diabetes. The growing insulin resistance produces a long gradual rise in blood glucose as the compensatory hyperinsulinemia prevents a more rapid ascent. For more than a decade, blood glucose stays relatively normal. In children and adolescents, this phase can be accelerated: some develop the disease in as little as twenty-one months.[3]

Visceral fat deposited in and around the organs[4] is the main contributor to high insulin resistance. The very first place this fat starts to accumulate, often before insulin resistance becomes noticeable, is the liver.

Fatty liver

The liver, as we've seen, lies at the nexus of food energy storage and production. After absorption through the intestines, portal circulation delivers nutrients directly to the liver. No wonder that, since body fat is essentially a method of food energy storage, diseases of fat storage involve the liver intimately.

Remember that all fats are not created equal. Excess dietary fat bypasses the liver and can be stored anywhere in the body. Fat carried under the skin (subcutaneous fat) contributes to overall weight and body mass index but has minimal health consequences. It is cosmetically undesirable but seems to be otherwise metabolically innocuous.

Excess dietary carbohydrates and protein are stored first in the liver as glycogen. Once glycogen stores are full, DNL converts glucose to fat, which can then be exported out of the liver to the rest of the body, including to fat stores in and around the abdominal organs. When DNL exceeds the export capacity of the liver, fat accumulates in the liver, where it contributes to central obesity and has dangerous health consequences. Too much sugar and insulin, over too long a period of time, leads to fatty liver.[5]

79

Eventually, the overfilled, fatty liver becomes unable to accept any more glucose and starts becoming insulin resistant. As seen previously, this insulin resistance is an overflow phenomenon. As shown in Figure 7.2, the cycle proceeds as follows:

1. Hyperinsulinemia causes fatty liver.
2. Fatty liver causes insulin resistance.
3. Insulin resistance leads to compensatory hyperinsulinemia.
4. Repeat cycle.

Figure 7.2. Hormonal obesity IV: High insulin → fatty liver → insulin resistance

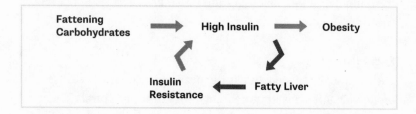

Fat inside the liver, rather than overall obesity, is the crucial stepping stone toward insulin resistance and diabetes. Fatty liver is associated at all stages of insulin resistance from obesity to prediabetes to full-blown diabetes. And that relationship holds in all racial groups and ethnicities.

Fatty liver is the clearest sign that hyperinsulinemia and insulin resistance are developing, and one of the earliest. Fatty liver precedes the clinical diagnosis of type 2 diabetes by ten years or more.[6] As the liver slowly accumulates fat it becomes increasingly insulin resistant. Fatty liver can be diagnosed by ultrasound, but an increased waist circumference or waist-to-height ratio is an important clue to its presence. Blood markers of liver damage also often mirror that slow rise, and this phase has been termed "the long, silent scream from the liver."

Two main types of fatty liver disease exist: alcohol-related liver disease and non-alcoholic fatty liver disease. The first is associated, as the name suggests, with drinking too much alcohol. Since most alcohol is metabolized solely in the liver, too much, too often forces the body to deal with the overflow. The result is fatty liver. But a lot of people who develop fatty liver disease and diabetes are not alcoholics, and it's only recently that scientists have begun to understand that connection.

Non-alcoholic fatty liver disease (NAFLD)

Dr. Alfred Fröhlich from the University of Vienna first began to unravel the neuro-hormonal basis of obesity in 1890. He described a young boy with the sudden onset of obesity who was eventually diagnosed with damage to the hypothalamus area of the brain, which resulted in intractable weight gain. This established this region as a key regulator of energy balance.

In rats, injury to the hypothalamic area of the brain could experimentally produce insatiable appetites and induce obesity. Researchers quickly noticed something else, too. All these obese animals shared characteristic liver damage, which was occasionally severe enough to progress to complete destruction. Genetically obese mice shared the same liver lesions. Strange, they thought. What does the liver have to do with obesity?

Dr. Samuel Zelman, a physician at the Veterans Administration Hospital in Topeka, Kansas, first made the connection in 1952.[7] Alcoholism was known to cause fatty liver, but he observed the disease in a hospital aide who drank, not alcohol, but more than twenty bottles of Coca-Cola a day! That obesity could cause similar liver damage by itself was completely unknown at that time. Zelman, aware of the data from experiments involving rats, spent the next few years tracking down twenty other obese, non-alcoholic patients with evidence of liver disease and found they unanimously preferred carbohydrate-rich diets.

Almost thirty years later, Dr. Jürgen Ludwig of the Mayo Clinic also described twenty patients with non-alcoholic fatty liver disease (NAFLD).[8] All these patients also suffered from obesity and obesity-associated diseases, such as diabetes. There was also varying evidence of liver damage. Those with NAFLD whose blood tests showed evidence of organ damage were said to have non-alcoholic steatohepatitis (NASH), a term derived from *steato,* which means "fat," and *hepatitis,* which means "inflammation of the liver." NASH is simply the more serious manifestation of NAFLD.

At the time of its discovery in 1980, Dr. Ludwig wrote that NAFLD spared doctors "the embarrassment (or worse) that may result from the ensuing verbal exchanges." In other words, the realization that fatty liver could occur without alcohol saved patients from their doctors' repeated accusations that they were lying about their alcohol intake. More importantly, the new recognition of NAFLD confirmed the extraordinarily close association between obesity, hyperinsulinemia/ insulin resistance, and fatty liver. Where you found one, you almost invariably found the others.

Obese individuals have five to fifteen times the rate of fatty liver. Up to 85 percent of type 2 diabetics have fatty liver.[9] Even without diabetes, those with insulin resistance alone have higher levels of liver fat.[10] NAFLD is estimated to affect at least two-thirds of those with obesity.[11] Moreover, the incidence of NAFLD in both children and adults has been rising at an alarming rate,[12] increasing in parallel with obesity and type 2 diabetes.

Hepatic steatosis, the deposition of fat in the liver, is consistently one of the most important markers of insulin resistance.[13] In obese children, rising levels of alanine transaminase (ALT), an important blood marker of liver damage,[14] is directly linked to insulin resistance and the development of type 2 diabetes. The severity of fatty liver correlates to prediabetes, insulin resistance, and impairment of beta cell function. Furthermore, NASH has become one of the leading causes of end stage liver disease, known as cirrhosis, and one of the top indications for liver transplant in the Western world. In North America, the prevalence of NASH is estimated at 23 percent of the entire population.[15]

This is a truly frightening epidemic. In the space of a single generation, non-alcoholic fatty liver disease has gone from being unnamed and completely unknown to being the commonest cause of abnormal liver enzymes and chronic liver disease in the Western world.[16] This is the Rocky Balboa of liver diseases.

Figure 7.3. Insulin resistance rises with liver fat[17]

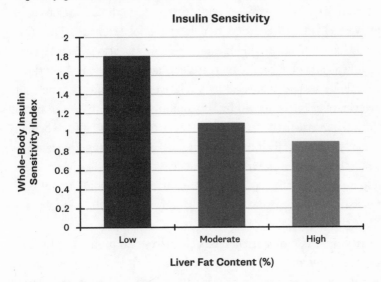

Insulin Sensitivity

(y-axis: Whole-Body Insulin Sensitivity Index; x-axis: Liver Fat Content (%), categories Low, Moderate, High)

Why some people have severe fatty infiltration of the liver without evidence of damage while others have minimal fat and severe damage remains unknown.

As the liver slowly accumulates fat, insulin resistance escalates in lockstep. In type 2 diabetic patients, a close correlation exists between the amount of liver fat and the insulin dose required,[18] reflecting greater insulin resistance. In short, the fattier the liver, the higher the insulin resistance. Therefore, to understand insulin resistance, we must first understand how fatty liver develops.

How fatty liver develops

83

Here's a startling fact: I can give you fatty liver. Actually, I can give *anybody* fatty liver. What's the scariest part? This crucial first step toward type 2 diabetes only takes three weeks!

Excessive glucose and insulin drives new fat production (DNL). If this occurs faster than the liver can export it out to the adipocytes (fat cells), fat accumulates in the liver. This condition can be achieved simply by overeating sugary snacks. Hey presto, fatty liver disease.

Researchers fed overweight volunteers an extra thousand calories of sugary snacks daily in addition to their regular food consumption.[19] This sounds like a lot, but it only means ingesting an extra two small bags of candy, a glass of juice, and two cans of Coca-Cola per day. After three weeks, body weight increased by a relatively insignificant 2 percent. However, liver fat increased by a whopping 27 percent, caused by an identical increase in the rate of DNL. This fatty liver was far from benign, as blood markers of liver damage increased by a similar 30 percent.

But all was not lost. When volunteers returned to their usual diets, their weight, liver fat, and markers of liver damage all completely reversed. A mere 4 percent decrease in body weight reduced their liver fat by 25 percent.

Fatty liver is *a completely reversible process*. Emptying the liver of its surplus glucose and dropping insulin levels returns the liver to normal. Hyperinsulinemia drives DNL, which is the primary determinant of fatty liver disease. Normalizing insulin levels reverses the fatty liver. Refined carbohydrates, which cause large increases in insulin, are far more sinister than dietary fat. High carbohydrate intake can increase DNL tenfold, whereas high fat consumption, with correspondingly low carbohydrate intake, does not change hepatic fat production noticeably.[20]

Specifically, the sugar fructose, rather than glucose, is the main culprit,[21] even though fructose does not produce much insulin response. The next chapter explains why in more detail. By contrast, in type 1 diabetes, insulin levels are extremely low, causing *decreased* liver fat.[22]

84 Producing fatty liver in animals is simple, too. The delicacy known as *foie gras* is the fatty liver of a duck or a goose. Geese naturally develop large fatty livers to store energy in preparation for the long migration ahead, but more than four thousand years ago the Egyptians developed

a technique known as *gavage*. Originally done by hand, this deliberate overfeeding is now administered using more modern and efficient methods. A large amount of high-starch corn mash is fed directly into the goose or duck's digestive system several times per day through a tube called an *embuc*. In just ten to fourteen days, the liver becomes fatty and enlarged.

Producing foie gras in animals and fatty liver in humans is basically the same process. Deliberate carbohydrate overfeeding provokes the high insulin levels necessary to develop fatty liver. In 1977, the *Dietary Guidelines for Americans* strongly advised people to eat less fat and more carbohydrates, such as bread and pasta. The result? Dramatically increased insulin levels. Little did we know that we were, in essence, making human foie gras.

Fatty liver is the harbinger of insulin resistance, but it is only the beginning. The fat within other organs, including the skeletal muscles and the pancreas,[23] also play a leading role in this disease.

Fatty muscle
Skeletal muscles are the large muscle groups, such as the biceps, triceps, quadriceps, trunk, and gluteal muscles, that we use to move our limbs voluntarily. This differentiates them from smooth muscles—muscles such as the heart or diaphragm—which are largely not under voluntary control. Skeletal muscles burn the bulk of the glucose available after meals and store their own supply of glycogen to provide quick bursts of energy. This muscle glycogen is not available for use by other organs of the body. Normally, little fat is found in skeletal muscle. Fat cells are specialized for fat storage; muscle cells are not.

With hyperinsulinemia and excess sugar, the liver creates new fat by DNL and distributes these triglycerides throughout the body. When adipocytes (fat storage cells) become overwhelmed, skeletal muscles also take up the fat, leading ultimately to fat deposits between muscle fibers. The technical term is intramyocyte lipid accumulation, but it could easily be called fatty muscle.

85

We can see this process of developing fatty muscle more clearly in farm-raised cattle, where the accumulation of fat between muscle fibers is called delicious! The streaks of fat are clearly visible as marbling—the intermingling of fat with lean muscle. As the meat cooks, the fat melts, making the beef more tender, moist, and flavorful, as it literally bastes itself. For this reason, well-marbled beef commands a premium price. Kobe beef, the ultra-premium Japanese delicacy, is prized for its high degree of marbling. The United States Department of Agriculture grades beef based on the degree of marbling. Prime beef, the highest and most expensive grade, has the most marbling.

Cattle ranchers know that marbling depends almost entirely on diet. Cows are ruminants, which means they normally eat grass and do not develop marbling. The result is a more flavorful but less tender steak. However, a grain-heavy diet increases the growth rate as well as the marbling. For this reason, many grass-fed cows are "finished" with a period of corn feeding to develop the desired fatty muscle, or marbling. Carbohydrate-heavy diets cause fatty muscle. It's no secret in cattle, and it works just as well in humans.

Fatty liver produces insulin resistance in the liver. In the same manner, fatty muscle produces insulin resistance in skeletal muscles. Hyperinsulinemia forces too much fat and glucose inside the skeletal muscles. They become completely full, so insulin cannot push any more inside. This is the same overflow phenomenon. Since the skeletal muscles are so large, they contribute significantly to overall insulin resistance in the body.[24]

Fat deposition in skeletal muscles, obesity, and severity of insulin resistance are closely related.[25] Muscles from obese subjects take up fatty acid at an equal rate to lean subjects but burn it at only half the speed, leading to greater accumulation of fat within the muscles. Weight loss can partially rectify this problem.

Why can't the muscle just burn off this fat? The answer lies in the biochemical process known as the Randle cycle.

The Randle cycle

Dr. Philip Randle first described the glucose–fatty acid, or Randle, cycle in 1963.[26] Working with isolated heart and skeletal muscle cell preparations, Randle demonstrated that cells burning glucose could not burn fat and vice versa. Furthermore, this phenomenon did not require the assistance of insulin or any other hormones. Your body simply cannot use both fuels simultaneously. You either burn sugar or fat, but not both.

Most cells can use fat directly for energy but certain key cells, notably the brain, cannot. During the fasting state, large organs such as the liver, heart, pancreas, and skeletal muscles burn fat to conserve what little glucose is available for the brain. This essential survival mechanism maximizes the time humans can survive without eating. Since the liver cannot produce enough new glucose by the process of gluconeogenesis for the entire body, the Randle cycle helps conserve glucose for where it is needed the most. The liver also produces ketone bodies from fat, which provides up to 75 percent of the brain's energy requirements, and further conserves glucose.

The body's ability to block the use of glucose by relying on fatty acids instead has also been called physiological insulin resistance. When the body is mostly burning fat, such as during very low–carbohydrate diets or fasting, it cannot burn glucose. Therefore, if you start to eat carbohydrates, the cells temporarily cannot handle the glucose load and your blood glucose levels rise. This phenomenon looks like insulin resistance but is not really the same mechanism at all. As insulin rises, the body switches to burning glucose and the blood glucose levels fall back.

The opposite is also true. When the body is burning glucose, it cannot burn fat, but saves stored fat for later consumption. The Randle cycle ensures the skeletal muscle cells cannot simply burn off the excess fat when they are fully saturated with glucose. They are burning glucose, not fat, so it accumulates. *Voilà!* Fatty muscle and insulin resistance.

Fatty muscle and fatty liver lead to rising insulin resistance, provoking the compensatory hyperinsulinemia that keeps blood glucose normal. But as we've seen, this cycle eventually leads to the development of more insulin resistance in a classic, self-reinforcing cycle. Over time, the insulin levels march relentlessly higher, as does the insulin resistance. Ultimately, something's gotta give. Enter phase 2.

PHASE 2: BETA CELL DYSFUNCTION

BLOOD GLUCOSE RISES quickly when the pancreatic beta cells responsible for insulin production cannot keep pace with rising insulin resistance. When this compensatory mechanism fails, it only takes one to two years before a diagnosis of full-blown type 2 diabetes. Over time, insulin production peaks and eventually starts to fall.[27] The progressive decline in insulin production is often called beta cell dysfunction, or sometimes pancreatic burnout. But what causes this burnout?

Many researchers suggest hyperglycemia destroys beta cells. But there's an obvious and insurmountable problem with this theory. As insulin resistance develops, blood glucose stays relatively controlled. Glucose doesn't rise significantly until *after* beta cells fail. The beta cell dysfunction causes the high blood glucose, not the other way around.

The prevailing hypothesis is that the beta cells are simply worn out from overproducing insulin for so long. Like a rickety old engine that has been revved too many times, the excessive chronic workload has caused irreversible damage. However, three main problems exist with this paradigm of chronic progressive scarring of the pancreas.

First, beta cell function has been proven to be fully reversible. Dr. Roy Taylor of Newcastle University in the U.K. demonstrated pancreatic function recovery with an ultra-low calorie diet.[28] The fact that weight loss can reverse type 2 diabetes also implies reversibility to the beta cell function. Simply, the beta cells are not burnt out.

Second, with excessive use, the body generally responds with increased, not decreased, function. If you exercise a muscle, it gets

88

stronger; it doesn't burn out. With overactive secretion, glands generally get larger, not smaller. If you think and study a lot, you increase your knowledge; your brain doesn't burn out. The same holds true for the insulin-producing cells. They should grow larger (hypertrophy), not smaller (atrophy).

Finally, beta cell burnout implies that damage occurs only due to longstanding excessive use. It takes many decades of overactivity to produce scarring and fibrosis. The rising epidemic of type 2 diabetes in children and adolescents clearly proves this concept false. With type 2 diabetes now being diagnosed in children as young as three years old, it is inconceivable that any part of their body has already burned out.

What causes the beta cell dysfunction? Since this defect naturally follows insulin resistance, Ockham's razor suggests that the beta cell dysfunction should share the same basic mechanism as the insulin resistance. Specifically, the problem is fatty infiltration of organs, and recent research has identified the likely culprit. During the first phase, fatty liver and fatty muscles create increased insulin resistance. In the second phase, fatty pancreas creates beta cell dysfunction. The pancreas is not burnt out; it is merely clogged with fat.

Fatty pancreas

Hyperinsulinemia causes fatty liver, and to relieve the backup, this newly created fat is exported out of the liver to other parts of the body. Some of it ends up in adipocytes, and some in the skeletal muscle. The pancreas also becomes heavily infiltrated with fat.

The relationship between pancreatic weight and total body weight was first noted in 1920. Pancreases from obese cadavers contained almost double the fat of lean cadavers.[29] By the 1960s, advances in non-invasive imaging allowed direct measurement of pancreatic fat and firmly established the connection between fatty pancreas, obesity, high triglycerides, and insulin resistance. Virtually all patients with fatty pancreas also had fatty liver.

Most importantly, fatty pancreas is clearly associated with type 2 diabetes.[30] Type 2 diabetic patients have more pancreatic and hepatic fat than nondiabetics.[31] The more fat found in the pancreas, the less insulin it secretes.[32] Simply put, fatty pancreas and fatty liver is the difference between a type 2 diabetic and a nondiabetic.

The difference is obvious during bariatric (weight-loss) surgery, which is used to reduce the size of the stomach or bypass the small intestine (more on this in Chapter 13). This surgery does not directly remove fat, like liposuction, which has no metabolic benefits.[33] Obese nondiabetics have a normal amount of pancreatic fat, which remains unchanged after surgery despite the weight loss.

Obese type 2 diabetics have excess pancreatic fat, but bariatric surgery reduces it and restores normal insulin-secreting ability. The result is successful reversal of type 2 diabetes within weeks of their surgery, even if they are still hundreds of kilograms overweight. The excess pancreatic fat is *only* found in type 2 diabetics. The pancreatic beta cells were clearly not burnt out; they were clogged with fat. The removal of only 0.6 grams of pancreatic fat successfully reverses type 2 diabetes. Eight weeks after bariatric surgery, liver fat also normalizes, as does insulin resistance.

Bariatric surgery is not the only method of achieving these benefits. Sudden severe caloric restriction in the COUNTERPOINT Study[34] decreased the amount of fat in the pancreas and re-established its ability to secrete insulin within weeks.

Ectopic fat, the accumulation of fat in places other than fat cells, plays a critical role in the development of insulin resistance. This includes fatty liver, fatty muscle, and fatty pancreas. Even in severely obese patients, insulin resistance does not develop in the absence of ectopic fat accumulation.[35] This fact explains how an estimated 20 percent of obese individuals may have no insulin resistance and normal metabolic profiles.[36] Conversely, normal-weight subjects may develop type 2 diabetes if the fat is deposited in the organs instead of in the fat cells. Fat inside fat cells is okay. Fat inside organs is not.

First noted in the 1950s,[37] visceral obesity, also called central obesity or abdominal obesity, is metabolically damaging. In the absence of insulin, these ectopic fat deposits, and hence insulin resistance, cannot develop.[38] Indeed, accumulated fat deposits melt away under conditions of sustained low insulin levels. Insulin is required to convert excess calories to fat and also to sustain it as fat.

Developing type 2 diabetes is not simply a function of increased body fat but the accumulation of *intra-organic fat*. The problem is not just the fat, it's the *ectopic* fat. Fatty liver and muscle drives the insulin resistance seen in the first phase of development of type 2 diabetes. Fatty pancreas drives the beta cell dysfunction seen in the second phase. The twin defects of type 2 diabetes include

- insulin resistance caused by fatty liver and fatty skeletal muscle, and
- beta cell dysfunction caused by fatty pancreas.

Importantly, these two fundamental defects are not caused by two completely different mechanisms. They are manifestations of the same essential problem: intra-organic fat accumulation driven by hyperinsulinemia, which is caused ultimately by excessive dietary glucose and fructose. Essentially, *too much sugar* causes type 2 diabetes. This answer is the simplest, most intuitive, and most correct. Ockham's razor cuts through the confusion.

THE DUAL CYCLES: A SUMMARY

TWO VICIOUS CYCLES sustain type 2 diabetes: the hepatic and the pancreatic. The hepatic cycle develops first. Excessive glucose and fructose ingestion leads to hyperinsulinemia, fatty liver, and then insulin resistance. The vicious cycle has begun. High insulin resistance further stimulates hyperinsulinemia, perpetuating the cycle. This dance goes around and around, gradually worsening each time.

Figure 7.4. The hepatic cycle (insulin resistance)

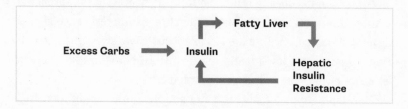

The hepatic cycle may continue for many years before the start of the pancreatic cycle. The fatty liver decompresses itself by exporting newly created fat as very low–density lipoprotein (VLDL) to other organs, including the skeletal muscles and pancreas. As fatty muscle develops, whole body insulin resistance worsens further. As the pancreas becomes clogged with fat, it becomes unable to secrete insulin normally. Insulin levels, previously high to offset the high blood glucose, begin to fall.

The loss of this compensation results in a rapid rise in blood glucose and, ultimately, the diagnosis of type 2 diabetes. Even though insulin drops, it stays maximally stimulated by the high blood glucose. This is the body's attempt to break this vicious cycle, as we shall soon discuss.

Figure 7.5. The pancreatic cycle (beta cell dysfunction)

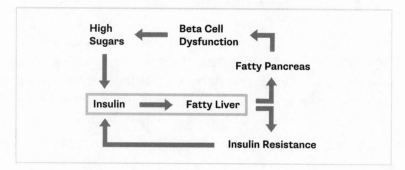

The hepatic (insulin resistance) cycle and the pancreatic (beta cell dysfunction) cycle together form the vicious twin cycles responsible for the development of type 2 diabetes. But they have the same underlying mechanism. Excessive insulin drives ectopic fat production and organ infiltration. The underlying cause of the entire cascade of type 2 diabetes is hyperinsulinemia. This is driven in turn by excessive dietary consumption of sugar, primarily glucose and fructose. Simply put, *type 2 diabetes is a disease entirely caused by too much sugar.* To understand fully, we need to consider the deadly effect of fructose.

8

THE FRUCTOSE-
INSULIN RESISTANCE
CONNECTION

....

I N 2009, DR. Robert Lustig, a pediatric endocrinologist at the University of California, San Francisco, delivered a ninety-minute lecture entitled "Sugar: The Bitter Truth.[1] The university posted it on YouTube as part of a medical education series. Then a funny thing happened. It went viral. It was not a humorous cat video. It was not a video of a toddler throwing a baseball into Dad's groin. It was a nutrition lecture filled with biochemistry and complicated graphs.

This particular lecture grabbed the world's attention and refused to let go. It has now been viewed more than seven million times. What was its attention-grabbing message? Sugar is toxic.

Dr. Lustig was not the first physician to warn about the dangers of eating too much sugar. In 1957, prominent British nutritionist Dr. John Yudkin warned that sugar played a prominent role in the growing incidence of heart disease. However, the world chose to follow Dr. Ancel Keys's condemnation of dietary fat instead. After leaving academic medicine, Yudkin wrote an eerily prescient book entitled *Pure, White and Deadly*,[2] but his warnings have largely gone unheeded.

The 1977 *Dietary Guidelines for Americans* distinctly warned the general public about the dangers of eating too much sugar, but this message got lost in the anti-fat hysteria that followed. Dietary fat was public enemy number one, and concerns about excess sugar faded like the last rays of sunset. Sugar consumption rose steadily from 1977 to 2000, paralleled by rising obesity rates. Ten years later, type 2 diabetes followed doggedly, like a bratty little brother.

Obesity alone does not fully explain the recent upsurge in diabetes. Some countries with low obesity rates have high diabetes rates, while the opposite is true, too.[3] Sri Lanka's obesity rates rose only 0.1 percent between 2000 and 2010, while diabetes rose from 3 percent to 11 percent. Over the same time period, in New Zealand, obesity rose from 23 percent to 34 percent while diabetes fell from 8 percent to 5 percent. Sugar consumption explains much of this discrepancy.

SUGAR BASICS

CARBOHYDRATES ARE SUGARS, either as single molecules (also called simple sugars or monosaccharides) or as chains of sugars (also called complex sugars or polysaccharides). Glucose and fructose are examples of single-sugar carbohydrates. Table sugar, known as sucrose, is a two-chain carbohydrate since it contains one molecule each of glucose and fructose.

Naturally occurring carbohydrates are said to be unrefined, or unprocessed. These include sugars found in fruit, vegetables, and raw grains. Refined carbohydrates have been processed: for example, wheat milled into flour; rice polished and hulled for easier steaming and boiling; corn treated with acids and enzymes to turn it into syrup.

As we saw in chapter 5, glucose is the primary sugar found in the blood. The terms blood sugar and blood glucose are used interchangeably. Every cell in the body can use glucose, and it circulates freely throughout the body. Muscle cells greedily import glucose from the blood for a quick energy boost. Certain cells, such as red blood cells, can *only* use glucose for energy.

95

Fructose is the sugar naturally found in fruit, and it is the sweetest-tasting naturally occurring carbohydrate. Only the liver can metabolize fructose, and this sugar does not circulate freely in the blood. The brain, muscles, and other tissues cannot use fructose directly for energy. Eating fructose does not appreciably change the body's blood glucose level, since they are different sugar molecules. Neither does fructose produce much insulin response directly.

Sucrose is composed of one molecule of glucose linked to one molecule of fructose, making it half glucose and half fructose. Chemically, high-fructose corn syrup is similar to sucrose, being composed of 55 percent fructose and 45 percent glucose. Pure fructose is generally not consumed directly, although it can be found as an ingredient in some processed foods.

Starches, the main carbohydrates in potatoes, wheat, corn, and rice, are long chains of glucose. Produced by plants, starches function as a store of energy. Sometimes they grow underground, as in root vegetables, and other times above ground, as in corn and wheat. By weight, starches are approximately 70 percent amylopectin and 30 percent amylose (both are types of glucose chains). Animals, including humans, chain glucose molecules together as glycogen instead of starch.

Once eaten, the chains of glucose in starches are broken down into individual glucose molecules and absorbed into the intestines. Refined carbohydrates, such as flour, are quickly digested, whereas unprocessed carbohydrates, such as beans, take much longer. As explained in chapter 4, the glycemic index reflects how much various carbohydrates raise blood glucose. Pure glucose causes the largest rise in blood glucose and is therefore given the maximal reference value of 100. All other foods are measured against this yardstick.

Other dietary sugars, like fructose or lactose (the sugar found in milk), do not raise blood glucose levels appreciably and therefore have correspondingly low glycemic index values. Since sucrose is half glucose and half fructose, it has an intermediate glycemic index. Only the glucose portion of sucrose raises blood glucose appreciably.

Fructose, which raises neither blood glucose nor insulin, was considered more benign than other sweeteners for many years. An all-natural sweetener found in fruit that didn't raise the glycemic index sure sounded healthy. But it had a hidden dark side that was not obvious for many decades. The toxicity of fructose was invisible when looking at the blood glucose; it only became apparent by looking at the slow accumulation of fat in the liver.

THE DOSE MAKES THE POISON

PARACELSUS (1493–1541), A Swiss-German physician who is considered the founder of modern toxicology, neatly summarized one of its most basic principles as "the dose makes the poison." That is, anything can be harmful in excessive amounts, even if it is typically considered beneficial. Oxygen can be toxic at high levels. Water, too, can be toxic at high levels. Fructose is no different.

Before the year 1900, the average person consumed 15 to 20 grams of fructose per day. All of it would have come from raw fruit, which contributes little fructose to our diet. An apple, for example, contains 7.6 grams of sugar per 100 grams; a grapefruit, just 1.2 grams. By World War II, sugar cane and sugar beets were farmed on large plantations, which made sucrose, the sugar processed from these plants, cheaper and more available than it had ever been. Yearly per capita consumption of fructose rose to 24 grams per day after the war and reached 37 grams per day by 1977.

In the 1960s, the development of high-fructose corn syrup (HFCS), a liquid-sugar equivalent of sucrose, became a game-changer. Processed from the river of cheap corn flowing out of the American Midwest, HFCS was much less expensive to produce than other forms of sugar. To increase profits, big food companies raced to replace sucrose with this cheaper substitute. Soon HFCS had found its way into almost every processed food imaginable: pizza sauces, soups, breads, cookies, cakes, ketchup, spreads.

97

Fructose intake skyrocketed. By 1994, the average person consumed 55 grams per day, or 10 percent of their calories. Fructose consumption finally peaked in the year 2000, by which time it had increased fivefold within the space of 100 years. Adolescents, in particular, were eating as much as 25 percent of their calories as added sugars, at 72.8 grams per day. Between the late 1970s and 2006, the per capita intake of sugar-sweetened beverages almost doubled to 141.7 kcal per day. Countries that use large amounts of HFCS have suffered a 20 percent increase in the prevalence of diabetes compared to those that do not. The United States, by the way, is the undisputed heavyweight champion of HFCS, with a per capita consumption of almost 55 pounds.[4] *The dose makes the poison.*

FRUCTOSE AND FATTY LIVER

FRUCTOSE IS EVEN more strongly linked to obesity and diabetes than glucose is. From a nutritional standpoint, neither fructose nor glucose contains essential nutrients. As a sweetener, both are similar. Yet fructose is particularly malevolent to human health compared to glucose due to the unique way the body metabolizes it.

Whereas every cell in the body can use glucose for energy, none can use fructose. Only the liver metabolizes fructose. Whereas excess glucose can be dispersed throughout the body for use as energy, fructose targets the liver like a guided missile.

When we eat large quantities of glucose, such as starches, these sugars circulate to every cell, helping disperse the load. Cells other than the liver metabolize 80 percent of the ingested glucose. At mealtimes, the heart, lungs, muscles, brain, and kidneys help themselves to this all-you-can-eat glucose buffet, leaving only 20 percent of it for the liver to mop up[5] and convert into glycogen for storage.

When we eat large quantities of fructose, on the other hand, it heads straight to the liver, since no other cells can use or metabolize it. Consider what this means for an average person weighing 170 pounds.

Sucrose provides equal amounts of glucose and fructose. Whereas all 170 pounds of the body metabolize the glucose, the 5-pound liver must valiantly metabolize the equivalent amount of fructose all on its own.

Moreover, the liver metabolizes fructose into glucose, lactose, and glycogen *without limitations*, so the more you eat, the more you metabolize. And because the refining process removes the protein, fiber, and fat naturally found in carbohydrates, the satiating effect of these constituents is lost. For example, 1000 calories of baked potato will make you quite full, but the same 1000 calories of sugary cola will not, despite that fact that both are mostly carbohydrate. However, one is unprocessed and the other is highly processed.

As a result, we digest refined carbohydrates such as HFCS faster, and because we don't feel full, we eat more of them and our blood glucose increases. When the limited glycogen stores are full, DNL changes the excess fructose directly into liver fat.

Fructose overfeeding can increase DNL fivefold,[6] and replacing glucose with a calorically equal amount of fructose increases liver fat by a massive 38 percent within only eight days. *This fatty liver plays a crucial role in the development of insulin resistance.* Fructose's propensity to cause fatty liver is unique among carbohydrates. Furthermore, *this harmful effect of fructose does not require high blood glucose or blood insulin levels to wreak its havoc.* Fructose functions as efficiently as a bullet train in causing fatty liver disease, which is only a short step away from insulin resistance.

Since fatty liver and the resultant insulin resistance is a key contributor to hyperinsulinemia and obesity, this means that fructose is far more dangerous than glucose. A back-of-the-envelope calculation shows that, for an average 170-pound person, fructose would be approximately 34 times (170 divided by 5) more likely to cause fatty liver and thus obesity and insulin resistance.

The way the body metabolizes ethanol (alcohol) is quite similar. Once ingested, tissues can only metabolize 20 percent of the alcohol, leaving 80 percent targeted straight to the liver.[7] The liver metabolizes it to acetaldehyde, which stimulates de novo lipogenesis, so alcohol, like fructose, easily becomes liver fat.[8] This explains the well-known effect of alcohol consumption in producing fatty liver disease.

Figure 8.1. Hormonal obesity V: Fructose, fatty liver, and insulin resistance

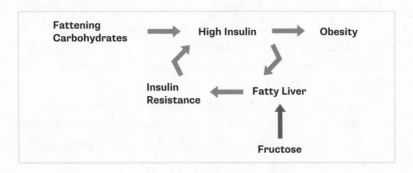

FRUCTOSE AND INSULIN RESISTANCE

THAT FRUCTOSE OVERFEEDING could experimentally provoke insulin resistance has been known since as far back as 1980. Healthy subjects overfed 1000 calories per day of fructose showed a 25 percent worsening of their insulin sensitivity after just seven days. Glucose overfeeding of subjects, by contrast, did not show any similar deterioration.[9]

A more recent study (2009) reinforced how easily fructose induces insulin resistance in healthy volunteers.[10] Subjects consumed 25 percent of their daily calories as Kool-Aid sweetened with either glucose or fructose. While this amount seems extreme, many people do consume this high a proportion of sugar in their diets. The fructose group—but not the glucose group—increased their insulin resistance so much that they would be clinically classified as prediabetics, a development that required only eight weeks of fructose overconsumption.

Remarkably, it only takes one week of excess fructose to cause insulin resistance. It only takes eight weeks to allow prediabetes to establish a beachhead. What happens after *decades* of high fructose consumption? The result is a diabetes disaster—precisely the one we are experiencing right now.

FRUCTOSE AND THE GLOBAL DIABETES EPIDEMIC

DATA FROM MORE than 175 nations links sugar intake inextricably to diabetes, independent of obesity. For example, Asian sugar consumption is rising at almost 5 percent per year, even as it has stabilized or fallen in North America. The result has been a tsunami of diabetes. In 2013, an estimated 11.6 percent of Chinese adults had type 2 diabetes.[11] Yet the Chinese being diagnosed with diabetes have an average body mass index of only 23.7, which is considered in the ideal range. By contrast, American diabetics average a body mass index of 28.7, well within the overweight category.

Consider that in 1980 only 1 percent of Chinese had type 2 diabetes. This situation presents an apparent paradox since the Chinese diet has traditionally been based upon white rice. Yet, despite such a high intake of refined carbohydrates, the Chinese have suffered little obesity or type 2 diabetes. The reason for this apparent protection is that they ate almost no sugar, as Figure 8.2 shows. Refined carbohydrates, such as white rice, are composed of long chains of glucose, whereas table sugar contains equal parts of glucose and fructose.

In the late 1990s, the INTERMAP study compared the diets of the U.K., U.S., Japan, and China.[12] Chinese sugar consumption has steadily increased since the time of that study, and diabetes rates have moved in lockstep. Combined with their original high-carbohydrate intake, the Chinese are facing their current diabetes disaster.

Figure 8.2. The traditional Chinese diet: High carbs, low sugar, no diabetes[13]

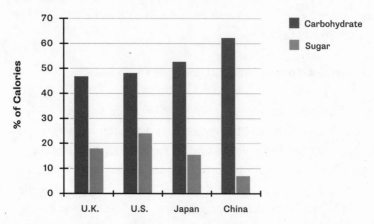

To a lesser extent, the same story has played out in the United States. Americans gradually switched from consuming their carbohydrates as grains to eating them as sugar in the form of corn syrup.[14] Consider Figure 8.3; when both grain and fructose intake began to rise in the late 1970s, the result was the start of an epidemic of obesity and type 2 diabetes.

Sugar is more fattening than any other refined carbohydrate, and leads specifically to type 2 diabetes. The prevalence of diabetes climbs 1.1 percent for every extra 150 sugar calories per person per day.[15] Each additional daily 12-oz serving of soda increases the risk of diabetes by 25 percent and the risk of metabolic syndrome by 20 percent.[16] No other food group—not dietary fat, not protein—shows any significant relationship to diabetes.

Diabetes correlates strongly to sugar, not other sources of calories. Fructose overconsumption directly stimulates fatty liver and leads directly to insulin resistance. Consumption of high-fructose corn syrup, which is chemically almost identical to sugar, also shows the same tight correlation to diabetes.[17]

Figure 8.3. Replacement of whole grain carbs with HFCS in the U.S.[18]

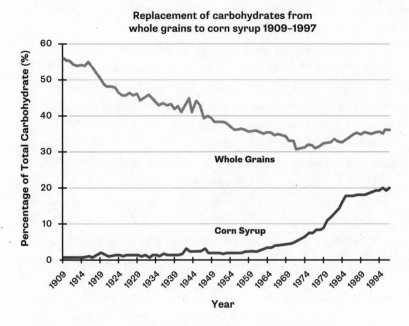

There is something sinister about overconsumption of fructose. What distinguishes sugar from other highly refined carbohydrates? What is the common link to disease? Fructose. Yes, Dr. Robert Lustig had it right. *The dose makes the poison*—and in the doses we are currently eating it, sugar is a toxin.

FRUCTOSE TOXICITY

FRUCTOSE IS PARTICULARLY toxic for several reasons. First, as we've seen, only the liver can metabolize it, so virtually all ingested fructose is stored as newly created fat. This excessive liver fat directly causes insulin resistance.

103

Second, the liver metabolizes fructose without limits. More ingested fructose leads to more hepatic DNL and more liver fat, independent of insulin. Fructose does little to activate natural satiety pathways that limit food intake, and no natural brakes exist to slow down the overproduction of new fat. This explains why you can still eat sweet desserts even after a full meal.

Third, fructose has no alternative runoff pathway. The liver stores excess glucose safely and easily as glycogen, breaking it back down into glucose when the body needs access to energy. On the other hand, the body cannot store fructose directly. When the body has enough energy to meet its actual needs, the liver metabolizes fructose into fat through a process that cannot be easily reversed. Therefore, the body can handle only small amounts of fructose. Remember, *the dose makes the poison.*

But this toxicity is not easily recognized. In the short term, fructose has few obvious health risks since it affects neither blood glucose nor insulin levels. Instead, it exerts its toxicity mainly through long-term effects on fatty liver and insulin resistance, which may take decades to manifest. Short-term studies, often focusing on insulin, blood glucose, and calories, miss this long-term effect, just as short-term studies of cigarette smoking miss the long-term cancer risk.

So sucrose or high-fructose corn syrup, both of which are roughly equal parts glucose and fructose, play a *dual* role in obesity and type 2 diabetes. More than simply empty calories, glucose is a refined carbohydrate that stimulates insulin production and, when consumed in large amounts, leads to fatty liver.

Overconsuming fructose, on the other hand, produces fatty liver and insulin resistance directly, without noticeably disturbing blood glucose or insulin. Fructose is many times more likely than glucose to cause fatty liver, setting off a vicious cycle. Insulin resistance leads to hyperinsulinemia, leading back to more insulin resistance.

Sugar, as both glucose and fructose, therefore stimulates insulin production in both the short term and the long term. In this way, sucrose is far more menacing than starches that contain only glucose, such as the amylopectin in flour. However, while the glycemic index makes the effect of glucose obvious, the effect of fructose is completely hidden, which has long led scientists to downplay the role of sugar in obesity.

A seemingly obvious solution is to replace fructose in the diet with artificial sweeteners. While the biochemistry of these compounds is far beyond the scope of this book, these agents are not a satisfactory solution to the fructose overload. The proof of the pudding is in the eating: we have used large and increasing amounts of these sweeteners in our diets and diabetes has not gone away. So we can debate why artificial sweeteners should work, but the bottom line is that they do not.

So when Dr. Lustig stepped onto that lonely stage in 2009 and declared that sugar was toxic, the world listened with rapt attention. This professor of endocrinology was telling us something we already, instinctively, knew to be true despite all the platitudes and the reassurances that sugar was not a problem: in sufficiently large amounts, sugar in any form is a toxin. *The dose makes the poison.*

THE METABOLIC
SYNDROME CONNECTION

....

THE IDENTIFICATION OF metabolic syndrome (MetS), originally termed Syndrome X, is one of the great medical advances of the past thirty years. The 2005 National Cholesterol Education Program (NCEP) Adult Treatment Program III (ATP III) defines metabolic syndrome as three of the following five conditions[1]:

1. Abdominal obesity, measured by waist circumference: men over 40 inches, women over 35 inches;
2. Low high-density lipoprotein (HDL): men less than 40 mg/dL or women less than 50 mg/dL or taking medication;
3. High triglycerides: over 150 mg/dL or taking medication;
4. High blood pressure: over 130 mmHg systolic (top number) or over 85 mmHg diastolic (bottom number) or taking medication;
5. Fasting blood glucose > 100 mg/dL or taking medication.

Metabolic syndrome affects almost one-third of the adult population of North America[2] and this linked group of problems increases the risk of heart disease by almost *300 percent*. Metabolic syndrome also increases the risk of stroke, cancer, NASH, PCOS, and obstructive sleep apnea. Even more worrisome, MetS is increasingly being diagnosed in our children.[3]

So what does metabolic syndrome have to do with diabetes? A lot, as it turns out.

UNDERSTANDING METABOLIC SYNDROME

IN 1988, DR. Gerald Reaven of Stanford University introduced the concept of a single syndrome in his Banting Medal address, one of the highest-profile academic lectures in all of diabetic medicine.[4] He called it Syndrome X to denote a single variable—then unknown—that caused this constellation of problems. But what was this X factor?

Our understanding of metabolic syndrome began in the 1950s, when researchers showed a close association between high levels of triglycerides and cardiovascular disease. To their surprise, hypertriglyceridemia was not caused by eating too much fat; instead, it resulted primarily from excess dietary carbohydrates and the subsequent hyperinsulinemia.[5]

Around the same time, early insulin assays confirmed that many people with relatively minor blood glucose elevations had severe hyperinsulinemia. This was understood as a compensatory mechanism in response to elevated insulin resistance. In 1963, Dr. Reaven observed that patients with heart attacks often had both high triglycerides and hyperinsulinemia,[6] firmly linking these two diseases.

Researchers noted a link between high blood pressure (hypertension) and hyperinsulinemia as early as 1966.[7] By 1985, research showed that much of essential hypertension, so called because the underlying cause remained unidentified, was also closely associated with high insulin levels.[8]

Remember that metabolic syndrome identifies patients with a shared group of risk factors that *all have a common origin*. High blood glucose, resulting from increased insulin resistance, central obesity, high blood pressure, and abnormal lipids all reflect a single underlying problem.[9] And each additional component of metabolic syndrome increases the risk of future cardiovascular disease. In fact, the major

107

diseases of the twenty-first century—heart disease, cancer, diabetes—have all been related to metabolic syndrome and its common cause, the X factor. That X factor, as it turns out, is hyperinsulinemia.[10]

It is worth noting that while obesity, as defined by BMI, is commonly associated with metabolic syndrome, MetS can also be found in approximately 25 percent of non-obese individuals with normal glucose tolerance levels. This emphasizes again that the problem is not obesity per se, but *abdominal* obesity. Similarly, high levels of low-density lipoprotein (LDL, or "bad" cholesterol) are pointedly *not* one of the criteria for developing metabolic syndrome. Despite the current obsession with lowering LDL cholesterol with statin medications, high LDL is not a component of the metabolic syndrome and may not have the same origins.

Recent research has supported and extended this concept of a single syndrome with a common cause. Let's see how this all develops.

FROM FATTY LIVER TO METABOLIC SYNDROME

AS WE'VE SEEN previously, the liver lies at the nexus of metabolism and nutrient flow, particularly for carbohydrates and proteins. Situated immediately downstream from the intestines, nutrients enter the blood in the portal circulation and pass directly to the liver. The major exception is dietary fat, which is absorbed directly into the lymphatic system as chylomicrons. These chylomicrons empty into the bloodstream without first passing through the liver.

As the major organ responsible for storing and distributing energy, the liver is naturally the main site of action of the hormone insulin. When carbohydrates and proteins are absorbed, the pancreas releases insulin. It travels in the portal vein, an expressway to the liver. Concentrations of glucose and insulin are often ten times higher in the blood of the portal system and liver than in the rest of the body.

Insulin promotes the storage of food energy for later use, a mechanism that has allowed us to survive the periods of famine inherent in human history. The liver prefers to store extra glucose in long glycogen chains since it is an easily accessible form of energy. However, there is limited space inside the liver for that glycogen. Think of a refrigerator. We can easily place food (glucose) into the refrigerator (glycogen) and take it out again. Once the glycogen stores are full, the liver must find a different storage form for the excess glucose. It transforms this glucose through de novo lipogenesis (DNL) into newly created molecules of triglycerides, also known as body fat.

Hypertriglyceridemia

These newly created triglycerides are made from the substrate glucose, *not* from dietary fat. This distinction is important because fats made by DNL are highly saturated. Eating dietary carbohydrates, *not* dietary saturated fat, increases saturated fat levels in the blood. Saturated fats in the *blood*, not the diet, are highly associated with heart disease.

When needed, the triglyceride molecule from body fat can be broken into three fatty acids, which most organs use directly for energy. The process of converting this fat to energy and back again is far more cumbersome than using glycogen. However, fat storage provides the unique advantage of unlimited storage space. Think of a chest freezer in your basement. Although it is more difficult to move food (triglycerides) into and out of your freezer (adipocytes, or fat cells), primarily because you have to move it farther, the size of the freezer allows you to store larger amounts. The basement also has enough space for a second or third freezer, if needed.

These two forms of storage fulfill different and complementary roles. The stored glucose, or glycogen (fridge), is easily accessible but limited in capacity. The stored body fat, or triglycerides (freezer), are hard to access but unlimited in capacity.

The two main activators of DNL are insulin and excessive dietary fructose. High dietary intake of carbohydrates—and to a lesser extent, protein—stimulates insulin secretion and provides the substrate for DNL. With DNL running at full production, large amounts of new fat

109

are created. Excessive DNL can overwhelm the export mechanism, resulting in abnormal retention of this new fat in the liver.[11] As you stuff more and more fat into the liver, it becomes noticeably engorged and can be diagnosed on ultrasound as fatty liver. But if the liver is not the appropriate place to store this new fat, where should it go?

First, you could try to burn it off for energy. However, with all the available glucose around after a meal, the body has no reason to burn the new fat. Imagine you have gone to Costco and bought waaayyy too much food to store in your refrigerator. One option is to eat it, but there's simply too much. If you cannot get rid of it, much of the food will be left on the counter where it will rot. So this option is not viable.

Your glycogen "fridge" is full, so the only remaining option is to export the newly created fat (excess food) somewhere else. This mechanism is known as the endogenous pathway of lipid transport. Essentially, triglycerides are packaged with special proteins to create very low–density lipoproteins (VLDL), which are released into the bloodstream to help decompress the congested liver.[12]

More dietary glucose and fructose means more DNL which means more VLDL must be released.[13, 14] This mass export of triglyceride-rich VLDL particles is the major reason for high plasma triglyceride levels,[15] which are detectable in all standard blood tests for cholesterol. Ultimately, eating too much glucose and too much fructose causes this hypertriglyceridemia.

Figure 9.1. Hormonal obesity VI: The effect of high triglycerides

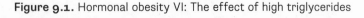

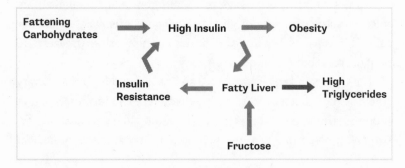

High-carbohydrate diets increase VLDL secretion and raise blood triglyceride levels by 30 to 40 percent.[16] Called carbohydrate-induced hypertriglyceridemia, this phenomenon can occur with as little as five days of high intake. Dr. Reaven showed that hyperinsulinemia and fructose shared responsibility for most of the rise in blood triglyceride levels.[17] Simply put, higher insulin levels and fructose ingestion produce higher blood triglyceride levels. There's just *too much sugar.*

Low high-density lipoproteins (HDL)

As VLDL particles circulate through the bloodstream, insulin stimulates the hormone lipoprotein lipase (LPL), which is found in the small blood vessels of muscles, adipocytes, and the heart. This LPL transports the triglycerides out of the blood into adipocytes for safe storage.

As VLDL releases its triglycerides, the particles become smaller and denser; now called VLDL remnants, the liver reabsorbs them. In turn, the liver releases these remnants back into the bloodstream as low-density lipoproteins (LDL), which are measured by standard blood cholesterol panels and are classically considered the "bad" cholesterol.

High blood triglycerides strongly and independently predict cardiovascular disease,[18] almost as powerfully as LDL, the marker that typically concerns doctors and patients most. Hypertriglyceridemia increases the risk of heart disease by as much as 61 percent,[19] and the average triglyceride level has been rising inexorably in the United States since 1976. An estimated 31 percent of adult Americans have elevated triglyceride levels,[20] though hypertriglyceridemia by itself is unlikely to cause heart disease since medications that lower triglycerides do not reduce the risk of cardiovascular disease.[21]

High levels of LDL are pointedly *not* one of the criteria for developing metabolic syndrome. Instead, the other cholesterol component of the metabolic syndrome is the high-density lipoproteins (HDL, the "good" cholesterol). The landmark Framingham studies established that low levels of HDL are strongly associated with heart disease[22] and predicts heart disease much more powerfully than LDL.

Low levels of HDL are found in close association with high levels of triglycerides: more than 50 percent of patients with low HDL also have high triglycerides. High levels of triglycerides activate the enzyme cholesterol ester transfer protein (CETP), which reduces HDL levels. Given this close association with triglycerides, it should be no surprise that low-carbohydrate diets raise HDL,[23] even independent of weight loss. As with triglycerides, low HDL does not cause heart disease, but is a powerful indicator.[24]

What is clear, however, is that the lipid profile typical of the metabolic syndrome—high triglycerides and low HDL—results from the excess of VLDL,[25] which ultimately stems from hyperinsulinemia, which ultimately stems from eating too much glucose and fructose. Again, *too much sugar.*

Figure 9.2. Hormonal obesity VII: Fatty liver → low HDL

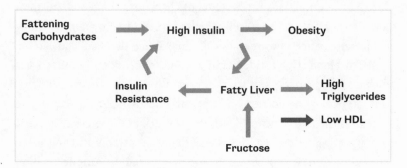

Abdominal obesity

The adipocytes get larger as they take up the triglycerides for storage. This is not particularly dangerous to our health since adipocytes are designed to store fat. But being too fat is dangerous from an evolutionary standpoint, because fat animals get eaten.

The adipocytes protect themselves against overexpansion by releasing the hormone leptin. This signals the hypothalamic area of the brain that we need to lose fat. We stop eating, insulin drops, and we lose

112

weight. In this way, obesity serves as the first line of defense against hyperinsulinemia.

Insulin encourages fat storage, whereas leptin strives to reduce it. If leptin proves more powerful, then weight is lost and fat mass decreases. This negative feedback loop should keep us at an ideal weight. So how do we become obese? This problem occurs when insulin stays too high for too long, which is typical in insulin resistance.

If you have too much body fat, leptin is released, which decreases food intake. Insulin should fall, and you should lose weight. In insulin-resistant states, insulin levels stay persistently high, which tells the body to keep storing fat. Leptin therefore stays persistently high too. As with all hormones, exposure creates resistance, so persistently high leptin creates the leptin resistance found in common obesity. It's a tug of war between insulin and leptin, and if you are eating too much sugar, ultimately, insulin wins.

Insulin allows glucose to move from the blood into the cells. Persistent hyperinsulinemia crams even more glucose into the liver, creating even more new fat. When hyperinsulinemia persists, the pedal-to-the-metal production of new fat overwhelms the adipocytes. Fat backs up, causing fatty liver. Fructose is directly converted to liver fat and leads to the next stage, insulin resistance.

If allowed to continue, the engorged liver will become distended and injured. The liver cell cannot safely handle any more glucose, yet insulin is still pushing really, really hard to shove more inside. The liver's only option is to refuse entry. This is known as insulin resistance, and it develops as the body's second line of defense against hyperinsulinemia.

The liver feverishly tries to relieve the fatty congestion by exporting triglycerides, and blood levels increase in a classic sign of metabolic syndrome. Ectopic fat accumulates in other organs, such as the pancreas, kidneys, heart, and muscle. The predominance of fat around the abdomen becomes noticeable as an increase in waist size, which can be described as a beer belly but more recently is being called a "wheat

113

belly." This abdominal, or visceral, fat is the most important predictor of metabolic syndrome.[26] Surgical removal of visceral fat reverses
insulin resistance,[27] whereas removal of subcutaneous fat has no such
metabolic benefits.[28]

High blood glucose

In addition to accumulating in the abdominal region, fat accumulates
within organs that are not designed to store it. Distention of the liver
and skeletal muscles with fat increases insulin resistance, even though
the pancreas increases insulin to keep blood glucose levels relatively
normal. But that's not the end of the story.

Ectopic fat clogs the pancreas and interferes with normal functioning, so insulin levels fall. When the fatty pancreas fails to produce
the compensatory hyperinsulinemia, blood glucose skyrockets and becomes symptomatic when it exceeds the renal threshold. Glucose spills
out into the urine, and the classic symptoms of diabetes—excessive
urination, thirst, and weight loss—appear.

High blood pressure (hypertension)

High blood pressure is often called "the silent killer" because there
are no symptoms, yet it contributes heavily to the development of
heart attacks and strokes. Most cases are called essential hypertension
because no specific cause can be found for its development; however,
hyperinsulinemia plays a key role.

Researchers first reported disproportionately high blood insulin concentration in hypertensive patients more than fifty years ago.[29]
Since then, multiple studies, such as the European Group Study of
Insulin Resistance,[30] have confirmed this relationship. High and rising
insulin levels doubled the risk of developing hypertension in those
who previously had normal blood pressure.[31] A complete review of all
available studies estimates that hyperinsulinemia increases the risk of
hypertension by 63 percent.[32]

Insulin increases blood pressure through multiple mechanisms.[33]
Insulin increases the cardiac output—the contractile force of the

heart[34]—and the volume of blood in circulation by enhancing the kidney's ability to reabsorb sodium (salt). In addition, insulin stimulates the secretion of anti-diuretic hormone, which helps the body to reabsorb water. Together, this salt and water retention mechanism increases blood volume and thus causes higher blood pressure. Insulin also constricts blood vessels, increasing the pressure inside.[35]

Figure 9.3. Hormonal obesity VIII: Hyperinsulinemia and hypertension

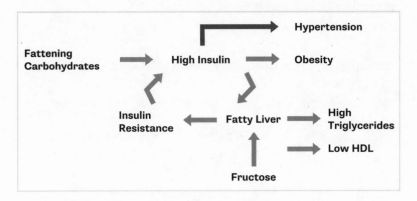

WHY METABOLIC SYNDROME MATTERS

EACH ADDITIONAL COMPONENT of metabolic syndrome—high triglycerides, low HDL, central obesity, high blood glucose, and high blood pressure—significantly increases the risk of all the modern metabolic diseases, such as heart attacks, strokes, peripheral vascular disease, type 2 diabetes, Alzheimer's disease, and cancer. These symptoms cluster together, but not every disease manifests in every person: one person may have low triglycerides, another person will have high blood sugars from insulin resistance, and yet another will have high blood pressure. But having one of these factors increases the likelihood of having the others because they all share the same root cause.

In a typical patient, gaining as little as 2 kilograms (4.4 pounds) of weight is the first detectable abnormality related to hyperinsulinemia/

115

insulin resistance, followed by low HDL cholesterol levels. High blood pressure, fatty liver, and high triglycerides emerge next, at roughly the same time. The very last symptom to appear is usually high blood glucose, which clinches the diagnosis of type 2 diabetes.

The West of Scotland study[36] confirmed that fatty liver and elevated triglycerides precede the diagnosis of type 2 diabetes. Fatty liver occurs early in metabolic syndrome. While virtually all patients with metabolic syndrome have fatty liver, the opposite is not true. Only a minority of patients with fatty liver have full-blown metabolic syndrome (see Figure 9.4).

Figure 9.4. Hormonal obesity IX: Full-blown metabolic syndrome

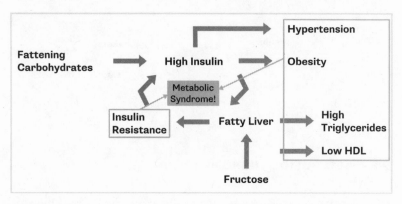

Insulin resistance and type 2 diabetes cannot cause metabolic syndrome because they are part of the syndrome. *Hyperinsulinemia* causes it. The very core of the problem is hyperinsulinemia from excessive fructose and glucose, but especially fructose intake. Metabolic syndrome, of which obesity and type 2 diabetes are a key part, are ultimately caused by—you guessed it—*too much sugar.*

116   Obesity, insulin resistance, and beta cell dysfunction are all protective mechanisms. Obesity tries to prevent DNL from overwhelming the liver by safely storing the newly created fat in the adipocytes. We know this because patients with a rare, genetic disorder called lipodystrophy, which is characterized by a lack of fat cells,[37] show all the manifestations

of metabolic syndrome—fatty liver, elevated triglycerides, and extremely high levels of insulin resistance—without the weight gain. In rodent models of lipodystrophy, transplanting adipocytes back into these fat-free mice completely cures metabolic syndrome.

Fat cells actually provide protection against metabolic syndrome rather than causing it. Why? Because without adipocytes, fat must be stored inside the organs, where it causes metabolic syndrome. If fat can be stored inside adipocytes instead, no metabolic damage results. Obesity is the first line of defense against the root problem of hyperinsulinemia/insulin resistance.

Similarly, insulin resistance is the body's attempt to prevent fat from amassing in the internal organs by preventing it from entering. The liver refuses to allow more glucose to enter because it is already overfilled, and the result is visible as insulin resistance, which represents a second protective mechanism.

The final line of defense lies in shutting down pancreatic production of insulin. Blood glucose rapidly rises above the renal threshold and causes all the classic symptoms of diabetes. *But this toxic load of glucose has been safely discharged out of the body, and is unable to cause further metabolic damage.* The core problems of too much glucose and insulin have been handled, but at the cost of symptomatic diabetes. The essential problem is too much sugar, and the body is desperately dumping it out in the urine.

All the conditions we thought were problems—obesity, insulin resistance, and beta cell dysfunction—are actually the body's *solutions* to a single root cause—*too much sugar.* And when we understand the root cause, the answer to all of these problems—and to type 2 diabetes—becomes immediately obvious. *We need to get rid of the sugar and lower insulin.*

If we fail to remove the problems of too much sugar, too much insulin, and ectopic fat, then the problem is chronic and progressive. When we treat the root cause, then type 2 diabetes, and indeed the entire metabolic syndrome, is a *completely reversible disease.*

BRUNO

Bruno, 75, had a thirty-year history of type 2 diabetes, which caused some eye and nerve damage as well as chronic kidney disease. He also suffered from gout, peripheral vascular disease, and high blood pressure. When we first met four years ago, he weighed 215 pounds and used 68 units of insulin daily.

Once he began the IDM program, Bruno started on a low-carbohydrate, healthy-fat diet with 36-hour fasts every other day. Within four weeks, he was able to stop taking insulin completely and has not required any since. This result still astounds him because he had been using insulin for over twenty years. In addition, he no longer needs any medication for blood pressure or cholesterol. His latest A1C is only 6.1%, which classifies him as prediabetic rather than diabetic.

Bruno adjusted quickly to his new diet and fasting regimen and finds it simple to follow, even several years later. He has maintained a 48-pound weight loss and a 24 cm reduction in waist size over these last four years.

RAVI

Ravi, now 40, was diagnosed with type 2 diabetes when he was only 28 years old. After starting on blood-glucose-lowering medications, he required higher and higher doses until he was finally prescribed insulin, which he was told he would need for life. In addition, he had developed high cholesterol and hypertension. He was taking 102 units of insulin daily, in addition to canagliflozin and metformin. Yet despite these huge doses of medication, his A1C was still 10.8%, which indicates that his blood glucose was completely out of control.

When Ravi entered the IDM program, he switched to a low-carbohydrate, healthy-fat diet and started fasting three times a week for 36 hours each time. Within two weeks, he was able to stop taking any insulin, and his blood glucose numbers were better than ever. Within two months, when his cholesterol and blood pressure had returned to normal, he stopped taking metformin and his doctor lowered his cholesterol and blood pressure medications to a quarter of their previous doses. In addition, he lost 23 pounds and his waist circumference decreased by 18 cm. Now, ten months into the program, he continues to take a single (non-insulin) medication, but his A1C is 7.4% and continues to improve.

(PART FOUR)

How Not to Treat
Type 2 Diabetes

INSULIN:
NOT THE ANSWER FOR
TYPE 2 DIABETES

....

THE CONVENTIONAL TREATMENT for both type 1 and type 2 diabetes has long been injection of exogenous (external) insulin. Human insulin, one of the great triumphs of modern pharmaceutical science, can be produced in a laboratory and packaged for convenient injection. For most of the early and mid-twentieth century, research focused on type 1 diabetes, which is caused by a severe lack of insulin. Without exogenous insulin replacement, cells cannot use glucose and they starve, leading to unrelenting weight loss and eventual death. This formerly fatal disease has become manageable, but injecting insulin comes with its own complications.

It is essential to match the insulin dose with the amount of food being eaten, especially carbohydrates, since complications arise when blood glucose goes too far outside the normal range. Underdosing causes high blood glucose (hyperglycemia) and overdosing causes low blood glucose (hypoglycemia). Mild hypoglycemic reactions cause patients to sweat and shake, but more severe reactions can include seizures, loss of consciousness, and death. In 2014, nearly 100,000 emergency room visits and 30,000 admissions to hospital were directly related to hypoglycemia.[1]

Extremely high blood glucose can cause diabetic ketoacidosis in type 1 diabetes and non-ketotic hyperosmolar coma in type 2 diabetes, but these complications are relatively uncommon. On the other hand, until the early 1990s it was unclear whether mildly elevated blood glucose was even all that dangerous. So for many decades, the standard medical practice was to keep the blood glucose levels slightly high, but below 10 mmol/L, the renal threshold for glucose. At this level, the kidneys completely reabsorb glucose so that none spills over into the urine, thereby avoiding the typical diabetic symptoms of excessive urination and thirst. And keeping the levels slightly above normal avoids both hypoglycemia and the symptoms of high blood glucose. In the past, this was considered an acceptable trade-off, as nobody had yet found definitive proof that this level was harmful. This point of view changed irrevocably in 1993.

INSULIN AND GLUCOTOXICITY

THE DIABETES CONTROL and Complications Trial (DCCT)[2]—a large, randomized, controlled trial of patients with type 1 diabetes carried out between 1983 and 1993—proved that intensive insulin therapy, including tight management of blood glucose levels, could have dramatic beneficial results. Close monitoring and multiple daily insulin injections to keep blood glucose levels as close to normal as possible could prevent the end-organ damage associated with hyperglycemia: diabetic eye disease decreased by 76 percent, kidney disease by 50 percent, and nerve damage by 60 percent.

In 2005, researchers published a follow-up study called the Epidemiology of Diabetes Interventions and Complications (EDIC).[3] They followed more than 90 percent of the original DCCT patients for up to seventeen years, and found that the intensive insulin treatment had reduced cardiovascular disease by an astonishing 42 percent. These two studies clearly established the paradigm of *glucotoxicity*—that high blood glucose is toxic in type 1 diabetes.

Figure 10.1. Intensive insulin therapy leads to major weight gain[4]

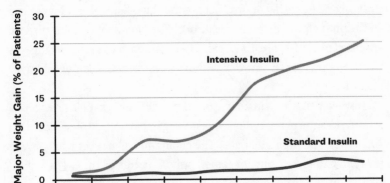

Some patients, however, paid a price. Hypoglycemic episodes during the DCCT study were three times more common in the intensive insulin group compared to those receiving standard treatment. Other patients experienced major weight gain. Over nine years, almost 30 percent of the subjects in that group gained a significant amount of weight, defined as an increase in body mass index of more than 5. This far exceeded the impact on those receiving conventional insulin therapy. One-quarter of that intensive treatment group had increased their body mass index from 24 (normal weight) to 31 (obese). Given the health consequences of obesity, this was no small concern. Other disquieting danger signs appeared, too. The weight gain was concentrated in the abdominal area, the central obesity known to be far more predictive of future cardiovascular disease. Other key risk factors, blood pressure and blood cholesterol, also increased.

Over time, weight, waist circumference, and insulin dosage continued to grow inexorably. Intensive insulin treatment had led to metabolic syndrome. Type 1 diabetic patients with the most weight gain also developed the highest coronary artery calcification (CAC) and carotid intimal medial thickness (CIMT) scores;[5] their high insulin dosage reliably predicted these measures of advanced atherosclerosis.[6] Heavy-handed dosing of insulin to reduce blood glucose had produced all the problems of excessive insulin: obesity, metabolic syndrome, and atherosclerosis. Despite these side effects, intensive insulin dosing was worth the risk for the proven cardiovascular benefits, *but only for type 1 diabetes.*

However, this glucotoxicity paradigm—the idea that elevated blood glucose was the primary cause of end-organ damage—was accepted for *both* type 1 and type 2 diabetes. The paradigm had not yet been proven for type 2 diabetes, but it seemed only a matter of time. The logical treatment was to give enough insulin or other medication to keep blood glucose normal. Even today, most doctors cling to this unproven treatment for type 2 diabetes like chewing gum clings to a boot sole. Does it work?

GLUCOTOXICITY AND TYPE 2 DIABETES

THE LANDMARK DCCT trial had established the paradigm of gluco-toxicity in type 1 diabetes. The United Kingdom Prospective Diabetes Study (UKPDS), started in the 1970s, was expected to prove the benefits of intensive blood glucose control in type 2 diabetes.[7] Researchers set out to determine two things about treatment: first, whether intensive glucose control could reduce complications, and second, whether there were differences among the different medications. The study randomly assigned almost 4000 newly diagnosed type 2 diabetic patients to either conventional or intensive treatments, using the available medications of the time: insulin, sulfonylureas (SUs), and metformin.

Published in 1998, the UKPDS results were stunning—stunningly bad, that is. Intensive treatment produced almost no measurable benefits. Sure, it successfully lowered the average blood glucose, but the higher dosages of medication resulted in more weight gain, by an average of 2.9 kg (6.4 pounds). In particular, those in the insulin group gained an average of 4 kg (8.8 pounds). Hypoglycemic reactions significantly increased, too, but these side effects were expected. Instead of mirroring the significant benefits of the DCCT trial, there was only some minor benefit in reducing eye disease. Ten years of tight blood glucose control produced no cardiovascular benefits: there were no fewer heart attacks or strokes. That discrepancy was shocking, but the story would get stranger still.

Metformin was considered separately in UKPDS sub-study 34,[8] which focused on overweight type 2 diabetic patients. Metformin lowered the hemoglobin A1C blood glucose level from 8.0 percent to 7.4 percent. This was good, but not as good as the results seen with the more powerful insulin and SU medications. Despite the mediocre blood glucose reductions, however, the cardiovascular results were spectacular. Metformin reduced diabetes-related death by a jaw-dropping 42 percent and the risk of heart attack by a whopping 39 percent, greatly outperforming the more powerful blood glucose–lowering agents. In other words, which specific type of diabetic medication you took made a huge difference. Metformin could save lives where the others could not, but its benefit had little or nothing to do with its blood glucose–lowering effect. The glucotoxicity paradigm, proven in type 1 diabetes, failed miserably in type 2.

The Cochrane group, a well-respected independent group of physicians and researchers, later estimated that glucose control was only responsible for a miniscule 5–15 percent of the risk of cardiovascular disease.[9] Yet that still wasn't the end of the story. Tired of all the controversy, and still confident of the glucotoxicity paradigm in type 2 diabetes, the National Institutes for Health in the United States funded the massive Action to Control Cardiac Risk in Diabetes (ACCORD) randomized study,[10] which began in 1999.

The ACCORD study recruited more than 10,000 type 2 adult diabetics across North America who were considered at high risk for heart attack and stroke. The trial was designed, in part, to test whether taking medications for intensive blood glucose control would reduce the risk of heart attack, stroke, death from cardiovascular disease, and other cardiovascular events.

One group of patients received standard treatment. The other group received high doses of medications and insulin to reduce blood glucose to as close to normal as possible. The first results from the ACCORD study were published in 2008 and proved that intensive medical therapy could reduce the A1C. Great. Did this make any difference to health? It sure did. *Intensive treatment was killing people.* Completely contrary to expectations, intensively treated patients were dying 22 percent faster than the standard treatment group, in spite of—*or perhaps because of*—the intervention. This equaled one extra death for every ninety-five patients treated. The study could not ethically be allowed to continue.

Many similar studies finished around the same time. The results of the randomized Action in Diabetes and Vascular Disease Controlled Evaluation (ADVANCE) trial, which looked at intensive blood glucose control and vascular disease in patients with type 2 diabetes, were published simultaneously with the ACCORD results.[11] Once again, this blood glucose–reducing strategy failed to deliver cardiovascular benefits; thankfully, it also failed to increase mortality. In contrast, blood pressure–lowering medications reduced cardiovascular disease, as expected. So certain medications did truly benefit type 2 diabetic patients, but those that reduced blood glucose did not.

Two further randomized controlled trials quickly followed to confirm these disappointing results. The Veterans Affairs' Diabetes Trial (VADT) found that intensive medical therapy produced no significant benefits to heart, kidney, or eye disease.[12] The Outcome Reduction with an Initial Glargine Intervention (ORIGIN) trial treated prediabetics with early initiation of insulin.[13] There was no reduction in heart disease, stroke, eye disease, peripheral vascular disease, or any measurable health benefits. The classic medications for type 2 diabetes, including insulin, metformin, TZDs, and SUs, had utterly failed to improve health.

The ACCORD, ADVANCE, and VADT trials all followed up with patients in the longer term and published extended results,[14] but these yielded little new information. All the trials agreed that intensive glucose control with medications did not save lives and had marginal, if any, benefits. Furthermore, there were serious side effects, including an increased risk of hypoglycemic reactions. The most obvious concern was the well-known propensity of SUs, TZDs, and insulin to cause weight gain in patients who were already obese, which could lead to cardiovascular problems down the line. Metformin, which does not raise insulin, does not cause obesity and this was the crucial difference.

Peer-reviewed commentary from 1999 reveals that concerns were already percolating about the real issue: exacerbating hyperinsulinemia in a patient who already had too much insulin. Dr. Richard Donnelly from the University of Nottingham, U.K., wrote, "The findings could also be interpreted as indicating that insulin and sulphonylureas are equally harmful in the obese, possibly as a consequence of hyperinsulinaemia."[15]

In type 1 diabetes, blood insulin is low, so replacing insulin is logical. In type 2, blood insulin is high, so giving more insulin seems problematic. After all, giving more alcohol to an alcoholic is not a winning strategy. Using heating blankets on a heat stroke victim is not a winning strategy. Treating sunburn by getting more sun is not a winning strategy. And giving more insulin to somebody with too much insulin is not a winning strategy. Logically, effectively treating type 2 diabetes requires an approach to lower *both* glucose and insulin, thereby minimizing both glucotoxicity and insulin toxicity.

INSULIN TOXICITY AND DOUBLE DIABETES

SINCE INTENSIVE GLUCOSE control using insulin caused weight gain and metabolic syndrome—hallmarks of hyperinsulinemia—in both type 1 and type 2 diabetics, and since type 1 diabetics produce none of their own insulin, this hyperinsulinemia could *only* be iatrogenic (caused by the treatment). Sound familiar? Hyperinsulinemia leads to insulin resistance. In type 1 diabetics, too much insulin causes the same exact problems found in type 2 diabetes. In other words, heavy dosing of insulin in type 1 diabetes creates type 2 diabetes. These patients essentially develop so-called double diabetes: they produce none of their own insulin and yet have all the problems of hyperinsulinemia due to exogenous injection. Too much insulin causes *insulin toxicity.*

Type 1 diabetics suffered all the same diseases as type 2 diabetics, but hyperglycemia was not the causal link. *Hyperinsulinemia* was the link. The European Diabetes Prospective Complications Study (EURO-DIAB study)[16] looked for factors that predicted risk of death for type 1 diabetics. It found that glucotoxicity, as measured by hemoglobin A1C, was *not* a significant risk factor. Instead, the most important modifiable risk factors were waist-to-hip ratio (a measure of visceral fat), blood pressure, and cholesterol—all markers of metabolic syndrome and hyperinsulinemia.

Many other studies confirmed the EURODIAB results. For example, the Golden Years Cohort Study[17] followed 400 patients with type 1 diabetes who lived for over fifty years with their disease. They had beaten the odds and survived. What was their secret? Well, it certainly was *not* tight blood glucose control. Their average A1C was 7.6 percent, with some as high as 8.5 to 9.0 percent, which is well above the standard recommended target of 7.0 percent. In fact, not a single Golden Years Cohort patient had an A1C in the normal range, ruling out glucotoxicity as a major player. The entire Golden Years Cohort of survivors had suboptimal blood glucose control and yet their health was excellent. The common factor was a *low insulin dosage.* Obesity, high blood pressure, and other manifestations of hyperinsulinemia were notably absent.

There are two toxicities at work here. Early on in type 1 diabetes, glucotoxicity is the main concern. In type 1 diabetics, this is caused by the body's inability to produce enough insulin. In type 2 diabetics, it's the effect of insulin resistance. But, in either type 1 or type 2, if you continually raise the dosage of insulin to lower blood glucose, you simply trade higher insulin toxicity for less glucotoxicity. And over time, insulin toxicity becomes the key determinant for survival because it leads to metabolic syndrome and its sequelae, cardiovascular disease and cancer. The optimal treatment strategy reduces *both* blood glucose *and* insulin simultaneously.

Type 2 DiabetesVille: A parable

Remember the Japanese subway pushers from chapter 6? How they were shoving more and more people into subway cars already bursting with passengers? And how ridiculous a solution that seems to dealing with the problem? That's exactly what happens when we use insulin to treat type 2 diabetes.

When I tell my patients with type 2 diabetes what's happening in their bodies, I use a slightly different analogy. Instead of cells in your body or passengers on a subway car, imagine you live on Liver Street in a town called DiabetesVille. Everybody is friendly and leaves their door open and unlocked. Three times a day, Mr. Insulin drives down the streets and delivers a small cup of glucose to each house for residents to enjoy. Life is going well, and everybody is happy.

Gradually, over time, Mr. Insulin comes around more and more often, and soon he's dropping off whole heaping buckets of glucose. He needs to empty his glucose truck every night, or he'll lose his job. For a while, you store the excess glucose in your house and life goes on. But finally your house is completely filled with glucose, which is starting to rot and stink. You try to reason with Mr. Insulin, but to no avail. Every house on every street has the same problem.

Now what do you do? Exasperated, you shout, "I don't want this toxic glucose! I've got too much already, and I don't want anymore." You lock the front door so Mr. Insulin can't shove any more toxic stuff into your house. A little glucose was fine, but this amount is getting ridiculous. *The dose makes the poison.* You are simply protecting your house by resisting Mr. Insulin's toxic glucose load. That's insulin resistance!

Mr. Insulin now finds it harder and harder to get rid of his glucose load and is worried he's going to get fired. So he asks his brothers to help. They break down your door and shovel in barrels of glucose—until you increase your front door's resistance with steel bars. It's a race between Mr. Insulin finding more Insulin henchmen, and you increasing resistance. More insulin leads to more resistance, and more resistance leads to more insulin.

With so much glucose stored inside the house, you turn it into fat, package it, and send it out to your friends on Pancreas Avenue, Skeletal Muscle Drive, and elsewhere. (In our cells at this point, the glucose has stimulated insulin and flooded the liver, which has activated DNL to transform this glucose into new molecules of fat. The excess fat is accumulating in the liver causing damage, so the engorged liver decompresses itself by moving this fat out to the pancreas, skeletal muscle, and around the abdominal organs. Meanwhile, insulin is still trying to force glucose inside, and the liver cells protect themselves by increasing insulin resistance.)

Back in DiabetesVille, all the doors have been triple-barred and guarded by dogs—big dogs. The Insulin brothers are now unable to deliver their huge glucose burden. Glucose is spilling over into the streets. Unsure what else to do, the specialist Dr. Endocrine steps in. He decides that the glucose is indeed toxic, and the streets must be cleared immediately.

Despite the hordes of Insulin clansmen prowling around, Dr. Endo decides that the best solution is to use even more insulin. He hires more Insulin thugs to shove more glucose into the reluctant houses, clearing off the streets. He gives himself a pat on the back. "Look," he says, "the streets are nice and clean."

132   But eventually the houses fill up again, and increase their resistance yet again. Even the extra Insulin cronies cannot shove any more glucose in. Does Dr. Endo get rid of some of the glucose? Does he stop glucose from coming into the city? No! He has only learned one

solution to every problem: give more insulin. To a man with a hammer, everything looks like a nail.

In our bodies, excessive sugar has led to too much insulin. Yet the currently accepted solution is to prescribe even more insulin. If insulin levels were already high, why would you want to give more? Instead of eliminating the sugar, insulin merely moves it around the body into all the organs. Higher insulin doses only create more insulin resistance. Even while the symptom of high blood glucose improves, the disease of type 2 diabetes worsens.

We accept that high blood glucose levels are harmful. But here's a question seldom asked. If this high glucose level were toxic in the blood, why wouldn't it also be toxic inside the cells? As glucose enters the cells faster than it can be used for energy, it accumulates inside the cell. The reason insulin resistance develops in all the organs and in all peoples of the world is precisely to shield against this toxic sugar load. It's a *good thing*, not a bad one.

Insulin doesn't actually eliminate glucose from the body; it merely shoves the excess glucose out of the blood and forces it into the cells, somewhere, anywhere: eyes, kidneys, nerves, heart. Over time, all the organs simply start rotting from too much glucose. Using medications like insulin to hide the blood glucose in the tissues of the body is ultimately destructive. The key to the proper treatment of type 2 diabetes is to get rid of the excess sugar, not just move it around the body. The problem is *both* too much glucose *and* too much insulin.

HYPERINSULINEMIA, INSULIN TOXICITY, AND DISEASE

HYPERINSULINEMIA WAS CONSIDERED a potential problem as far back as 1924,[18] but only more recently have researchers started to look closely at the data, and the evidence is everywhere.[19] Too much insulin leads to insulin toxicity, which is strongly associated with many diseases.[20]

Atherosclerosis and cardiovascular disease

While type 2 diabetes is associated with numerous complications, including nerve, kidney, and eye damage, the morbidity and mortality associated with cardiovascular diseases is the most important.[21] Simply put, most diabetic patients die of cardiovascular disease. As early as 1949, animal studies demonstrated that insulin treatment causes early atherosclerosis, also called hardening of the arteries, which is a precursor to heart attacks, strokes, and peripheral vascular disease. Insulin facilitates every single step along the inflammatory pathway that marks the progression of the disease, including initiation, inflammation, foam cell (fat-laden cell) formation, fibrous plaque formation, and advanced lesions.[22] Moreover, fibrous plaque contains insulin receptors,[23] and insulin stimulates the growth of plaque, which accelerates the atherosclerosis and substantially raises the risk of cardiovascular disease. Experimentally, these same studies showed that preventing the excessive insulin could reverse the condition.[24]

If you are not on diabetes medications, the risk of heart disease increases with the degree of hyperglycemia.[25] Insulin lowers blood glucose, so it has always been assumed it would protect against disease. But that is only true if glucotoxicity causes the heart disease, which it does not. What has not generally been appreciated is that, if you are not on diabetes medications, the degree of hyperglycemia reflects the severity of diabetes. Trading insulin toxicity for glucotoxicity is not obviously beneficial.

The UK General Practice Database identified more than 84,000 newly diagnosed diabetics between 2000 and 2010.[26] Treatment with insulin did not lower heart disease risk; rather, it more than doubled the risk of death. The same held true for heart attacks, strokes, cancer, and kidney disease. Insulin could reduce blood glucose but not heart disease or death.[27] Patients with an A1C blood glucose level of 6.0 percent, which was considered excellent control, fared just as poorly as those patients with an A1C of 10.5 percent, which is considered uncontrolled diabetes.[28] Ultimately, heavy-handed use of insulin could reduce glucotoxicity, but only at the expense of insulin toxicity. As in type 1 diabetes, high insulin doses were not good; they were bad.

Figure 10.2. Insulin use and increased risk of mortality in type 2 diabetes[29]

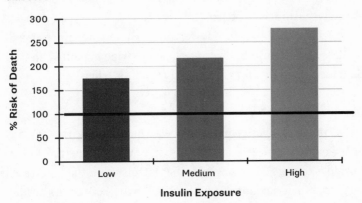

These results were not new. Reviews of large population databases, such as the 1996 Quebec Cardiovascular Study, established hyperinsulinemia as a prime risk factor for heart disease.[30] In Saskatchewan, Canada, a review of more than twelve thousand newly diagnosed diabetic patients found a "significant and graded association between mortality risk and insulin exposure level."[31] It wasn't a trivial effect, either. The high-insulin group had a 279 percent higher risk of death compared to those that did not use insulin. Treating type 2 diabetes with insulin was not good; it was bad. Simply put, the higher the insulin dose, the higher the risk of dying.

Moreover, the longer the treatment time with insulin, the greater the risk of cardiovascular disease.[32] A 2011 study showed that *both* low and high blood glucose carried excess risk of death, again reflecting the dual toxicities of glucose and insulin. Once again, insulin use was associated with a mind-boggling 265 percent increased risk of death.[33]

A Cardiff University review of almost 10 percent of the U.K. population from 2004 to 2015 found that *lower* A1C was associated with

135

elevated mortality risk, driven mainly by a 53 percent increased risk with the use of insulin.[34] In this study, no other medication increased the risk of death. A Dutch database associated high daily insulin doses with three times the cardiovascular risk.[35] In heart failure patients, insulin use is associated with more than four times the risk of death.[36]

Excessive insulin is toxic, particularly in a setting of type 2 diabetes, where baseline insulin is already very high. Giving more insulin will lower the blood glucose, but worsen the underlying hyperinsulinemia. Trading insulin toxicity for glucotoxicity is not beneficial.

Cancer

Diabetes, as well as obesity and prediabetes, increases the risk of many different types of cancer, including breast, colon, endometrial, kidney, and bladder cancers.[37] This suggests that factors other than increased blood glucose play a major role in the development of cancers, further disproving the glucotoxicity paradigm as the major cause of disease.[38]

Insulin, a hormone well known to promote growth, can drive tumor growth, and women with the highest insulin levels carry a 2.4-fold higher risk of breast cancer.[39] Obesity may be a contributing factor, but hyperinsulinemia is associated with an increased risk of cancer, independent of weight. Lean and overweight women, when matched for insulin level, exhibit the same risk of breast cancer.

The intimate link between insulin and cancer is reinforced by the discovery of a single mutation in the PTEN oncogene that significantly increases the risk of cancer.[40] What's the connection? This mutation increases the insulin effect. It lowers the blood glucose and reduces the risk of diabetes, but increases the risk of obesity and cancer.

Similarly, medications that raise insulin toxicity are associated with higher rates of cancer. Insulin use increases the risk of colon cancer by approximately 20 percent per year of therapy.[41] The UK General Practice Database revealed that insulin increased the risk of cancer by 42 percent compared with a glucose-lowering drug that did not raise insulin.[42] And a review of the newly diagnosed diabetics in the Saskatchewan population disclosed that use of insulin raised the risk of cancer by 90 percent.[43]

It's simple to understand why high insulin levels should favor cancer cell growth. First, insulin is a known hormonal growth factor. Second, cancer cells are highly metabolically active and need large supplies of glucose to proliferate. Insulin increases the risk of cancer, and once cancer has been established, high blood glucose enables it to grow faster.

ORAL HYPOGLYCEMICS:
NOT THE ANSWER

. . . .

A S OF 2012, more than 50 percent of the American population has diabetes or prediabetes.[1] This stunning statistic means more people in the United States have prediabetes or diabetes than not. It's the new normal. It's also made selling insulin and insulin-like drugs the money-making opportunity of a lifetime, which may explain why it continues to be prescribed for prediabetics and type 2 diabetics when it doesn't make sense.

In 2008, a joint statement released by the American College of Endocrinology and the American Association of Clinical Endocrinologists encouraged physicians to consider drug treatment of prediabetic patients despite the fact that no drug had yet been approved by the U.S. Food and Drug Administration.[2]

In 2010, the definition of type 2 diabetes was broadened, ostensibly to help with early diagnosis and treatment. It is perhaps no coincidence that nine of the fourteen outside experts on the panel that made this recommendation worked in various capacities with the giant pharmaceutical companies that made diabetes medications and stood directly in the path of an unending torrent of money. In the lead-up to this decision, individual members received millions of dollars and the American Diabetes Association itself reaped more than $7 million in 2004 alone from its pharmaceutical "partners."[3]

When Dr. Banting discovered insulin in 1921, he licenced the drug to pharmaceutical companies without a patent because he fervently believed this life-saving miracle should be made available to everybody who needed it. Yet, insulin—now available in many different formulations—is estimated to have cost the U.S. health care system $6 billion in 2012,[4] driven in part by steep price increases. Between 2010 and 2015, these newer insulins increased in price from 168 to 325 percent. In 2013, Lantus, a long-acting form of insulin, earned $7.6 billion, making it the world's bestselling diabetes drug. Various other insulins took another six of the top ten spots on that list.

Between 2004 and 2013, no less than thirty new diabetes drugs came to market. Despite several setbacks, by 2015 sales of diabetes drugs had reached $23 billion, which is more than the combined revenue of the National Football League, Major League Baseball, and the National Basketball Association.[5]

Figure 11.1. Increasing variety of diabetic medications[6]

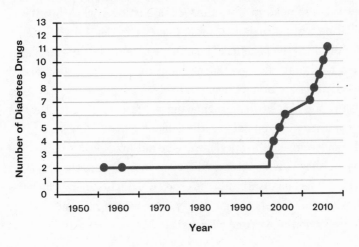

The focus of treatment of type 2 diabetes has always been to lower blood glucose because it is *associated* with better health outcomes. Every 1 percent increase in the hemoglobin A1C is associated with an 18 percent increase in risk of cardiovascular events, 12 to 14 percent increase in the risk of death, and 37 percent increase in risk of eye disease or kidney disease.[7]

But correlation is not causation. Lowering blood glucose with medications, as opposed to diet and lifestyle, is not necessarily beneficial. Consider two type 2 diabetic patients with an identical A1C of 6.5 percent. One takes no medications and the other uses 200 units of insulin daily. These might seem like identical situations, but they're not. The first situation reflects mild diabetes while the other reflects severe diabetes. The use of insulin does not change severe type 2 diabetes into mild type 2 diabetes. The cardiovascular risks are completely different. Indeed, insulin may not have any benefits at all.

No evidence exists that these newer insulins are any more effective than the original. Indeed, health outcomes for type 2 diabetes have only worsened even as these newer insulins have become more widely prescribed. And exogenous insulin injections are no longer just for type 1 diabetes. Almost one-third of diabetics in the United States currently use some form of insulin.[8] This statistic is slightly horrifying, considering that 90 to 95 percent of diabetes in the United States is type 2, for which the benefits of insulin are highly questionable.

In fact, other medications are available for type 2 diabetes. Several classes of drugs are or have been available through the years, and are still being prescribed to a bigger and bigger group of patients. Despite their popularity among doctors, these blood glucose–lowering pills— oral hypoglycemics in medicalspeak—are not long-term solutions to diabetes, either. I divide these medications into three categories based upon their effect on insulin and thus body weight. In general, the more they raise insulin levels, the more they cause weight gain and many of the complications associated with diabetes.

MEDICATIONS THAT CAUSE WEIGHT GAIN

Sulfonylureas (SUs)

Sulfonylureas stimulate the pancreas to produce more insulin, thereby effectively reducing blood sugars. The sulfonylurea (SU) drug class was discovered in 1942 and has been widely prescribed since then. By 1984, more powerful second-generation SUs had been introduced in the United States. The most commonly used drugs in this class include glyburide, glipizide, and glicizide.

In its research on type 2 diabetes, the United Kingdom Prospective Diabetes Study (UKPDS; see chapter 10) demonstrated that intensive treatment with the SU class of drugs produced almost no benefits in controlling the long-term complications of diabetes. Of particular concern was that exacerbating weight gain in already obese patients could lead to cardiovascular problems down the line. Extended follow-up of the original UKPDS study showed only mild cardiovascular benefits: the death rate was reduced by 13 percent.[9] The paradigm of glucotoxicity was established for type 2 diabetes, but only barely. Blood glucose–lowering medications had marginal benefits that took twenty years to become apparent. The risk associated with increasing insulin, with its accompanying weight gain, could barely offset the benefit of lowering glucose.

Further studies have borne out these concerns. A 2012 review of more than 250,000 newly diagnosed type 2 diabetics in the Veterans Affairs database across the United States showed that starting treatment with SUs instead of metformin carries a 21 percent higher risk of cardiovascular disease.[10] Studies from the U.K. and elsewhere estimate the use of SUs increases the risk of heart attack or death by 40 to 60 percent.[11] Furthermore, these risks increase in a dose-dependent manner.[12] That is, the higher the dose of SU, the greater the cardiovascular risk.

A 2012 randomized, controlled trial, the gold standard of evidence-based medicine, confirmed that initial therapy with SUs compared to metformin increases the risk of vascular disease by 40 percent[13] *despite equal blood glucose control*. The importance of this study cannot be underestimated. Two drugs that control blood glucose equally could have widely divergent effects on cardiovascular health. The main difference? One stimulates insulin and causes weight gain whereas the other does not. Glucotoxicity is equal, so the difference is the insulin toxicity of SUs.

Thiazolidinediones (TZDs)

During the 1980s and 1990s, drug companies did not develop a single new oral hypoglycemic agent because the number of patients using them was too small and the benefit was dubious. But the growing number of diabetics and prediabetics changed the economics of diabetic medications completely. In 1999, the Federal Drug Administration (FDA) approved the first new diabetes drug class in more than a decade, the thiazolidinediones (TZDs). These drugs bind to receptors in the fat cells, making them more sensitive to insulin and thereby amplifying insulin's effects. So TZDs such as rosiglitazone, sold under the brand name Avandia, and pioglitazone, sold as Actos, lower blood glucose but do not raise insulin levels; instead, they help the body use the available insulin more effectively.

Predictably, research showed TZDs' magnifying effect was both positive and negative. Blood glucose was lowered, but patients could reliably expect to gain 3 to 4 kilograms (6.6 to 8.8 pounds) of fat, as insulin is a key driver of weight gain. They also retained fluid, typically around the ankles but sometimes in the lungs, which caused shortness of breath and congestive heart failure. These setbacks were mild, but worse was still to come.

By 2007, the influential *New England Journal of Medicine* reported that rosiglitazone unexpectedly increased the risk of heart attacks.[14] The FDA hastily convened an advisory board of independent experts that same year;[15] similar deliberations took place in Europe. The FDA investigated concerns of data tampering in the Residential Environment and Coronary Heart Disease (RECORD) study, one of the largest trials that had "proved" the safety of rosiglitazone, and eventually concluded that the concerns about heart disease were well placed.[16] Rosiglitazone was associated with a 25 percent higher risk of heart attack.

By 2011, Europe, the U.K., India, New Zealand, and South Africa had all banned the use of rosiglitazone, though the FDA continued to allow its sale in the United States with a warning label for patients. These concerns devastated sales. Doctors stopped prescribing the medication, patients refused to take it, and by 2012, sales had fallen to a paltry $9.5 million.

The debacle left some beneficial policy changes in its wake. All diabetes medications henceforth were required to conduct large-scale safety trials to safeguard the public interest. Dr. Clifford Rosen, the chairperson of that FDA committee, clearly identified the key problem. New drugs were approved based solely on their ability to lower blood glucose, under the unproven assumption that this effect would reduce the cardiovascular burden. However, the evidence to date, including the UKPDS, ACCORD, ADVANCE, VADT, and ORIGIN studies, had failed to confirm these theorized benefits. Lowering blood glucose had little to do with protecting against the organ damage of type 2 diabetes.

A second TZD, pioglitazone, faced its own concerns about bladder cancer. Compared to other diabetes medications, the use of pioglitazone is associated with a 63 percent increased risk of bladder cancer.[17] The risk rises with longer duration of use and higher dosages.

The known side effects of weight gain and fluid retention were enough to give physicians pause, but these new concerns about cardiovascular and cancer risks effectively sealed the fate of the TZD drug class. In North America, they are very rarely prescribed and usage has effectively ceased.

MEDICATIONS THAT ARE WEIGHT NEUTRAL

Metformin

Metformin, the most powerful of the biguanide class of medications, was discovered shortly after insulin and described in the scientific literature in 1922. By 1929, its sugar-lowering effect was noted in animal studies, but it was not until 1957 that it was first used in humans for the treatment of diabetes. Biguanides work by blocking gluconeogenesis and thereby preventing the liver from producing glucose. This effect lowers the risk of hypoglycemia and weight gain because it does not increase insulin levels in the body.

Metformin entered the British National Formulary in 1958 and was introduced in Canada in 1972. The FDA did not approve it in the United States until 1994 due to concerns about an extremely rare side effect called lactic acidosis. However, given the powerful lifesaving effect demonstrated in the UKPDS compared to other comparable diabetes drugs, the benefits are felt to be well worth the risk and it has become the most widely prescribed diabetes drug in the world.

Since metformin does not raise insulin, it does not cause obesity and therefore does not worsen diabetes. So metformin sounds pretty good. The problem is that metformin (and other biguanides) does not take away the root cause of the illness—that is, they do not rid the body of excess sugar. Remember, hyperinsulinemia causes type 2 diabetes. While these drugs target blood glucose, they do little to relieve the underlying hyperinsulinemia. They take care of the symptom but, since they do not eliminate the cause, insulin resistance continues to rise and diabetes is managed but not eliminated.

Clinically, this is obvious. Once started on metformin, it is highly unlikely that one will ever be able to stop it without intensive lifestyle changes. Therefore, metformin may manage the disease for a while, but eventually, the patient will require higher and higher doses. The underlying disease process continues progressing, solemn as a clergyman.

Dipeptidyl peptidase-4 (DPP-4) inhibitors

In 2006, the FDA approved a new class of medications called the dipeptidyl peptidase-4 (DPP-4) inhibitors. These drugs are designed to lower blood glucose by blocking the breakdown of incretins, which are hormones released in the stomach that increase insulin secretion in response to food. High incretin levels stimulate insulin release; however, this insulin response is not sustained and therefore these drugs do not cause weight gain. The risk of hypoglycemia is also low.

Hopes were high for this new class of medication, but a study completed in 2013, called the SAVOR study[18] (Saxagliptin Assessment Of Vascular Outcomes Recorded In Patients With Diabetes Mellitus), along with 2015's Trial Evaluating Cardiovascular Outcomes with Sitagliptin (TECOS) study,[19] soon dashed these hopes. The FDA mandated both randomized controlled trials after the rosiglitazone debacle and neither found safety concerns with the long-term use of these medications. However, neither were there any protective effects against cardiovascular diseases. These medications effectively lowered blood glucose but did not reduce heart attacks or strokes. Once again, the glucotoxicity paradigm was proven false. Yes, you could reduce blood glucose, but, no, you were not any healthier for it.

In spite of that, the fact that these medications were at least not killing people was apparently a good enough reason to prescribe them. In 2015, the top DPP-4 inhibitor, sitagliptin, raked in $3.86 billion, enough to rank it as the second bestselling diabetes drug in the world, trailing only Lantus, a long-acting form of insulin.[20]

MEDICATIONS THAT CAUSE WEIGHT LOSS

Sodium-glucose cotransporter 2 (SGLT2) inhibitors

The newest class of medications, called sodium-glucose cotransporter 2 (SGLT2) inhibitors, block glucose reabsorption in the kidney, allowing glucose to escape in the urine, which replicates the protective mechanism used by the body during severe hyperglycemia. What happens if you don't block this protective mechanism, but enhance it?

Where the classic diabetes drugs increase insulin, the SGLT2 inhibitors lower it[21] by forcing the excretion of glucose outside the body. The result is lower blood glucose, but also lower body weight, blood pressure, and markers of arterial stiffness.[22] As the root cause of diabesity

145

is hyperinsulinemia, here, at long last, was a drug that effectively lowered insulin. Would this finally translate into proven cardiovascular benefits?

It wasn't just a home run; it was a grand slam. A 2015 study called the EMPA-REG study (Empagliflozin: Cardiovascular (CV) Outcomes and Mortality in Patients with Type 2 Diabetes Mellitus)[23] revealed that the SLGT2s reduced the risk of death by an incredible 38 percent. The good news did not stop there. It reduced the risk of progression of kidney disease by almost 40 percent and the need for dialysis by a stunning 55 percent.[24] The elusive cardiovascular and renal benefits that virtually every previous study had failed to deliver were finally found.

Tellingly, the blood glucose–lowering effect was very modest. The A1C only dropped by 0.47 percent, far less than almost every other medication currently in use, but the benefits were far greater. This result once again underscored that glucotoxicity is a minor-league player. The SGLT2 inhibitors simultaneously lowered both insulin toxicity and glucotoxicity, and the results were nothing short of amazing.

Weight loss is one of the most noticeable side benefits of this class of medication. Not only did patients lose weight, unlike virtually every other dietary trial, they kept the weight off even after the two years. Canagliflozin, for example, helped patients lose an extra 2.9 kg of body weight and keep it off.[25]

The main side effect of this class of medications is the increased risk of urinary tract infections and yeast infections due to increased urinary glucose concentration. However, these infections were generally mild and treatable. The most serious side effect was an increased risk of ketoacidosis. The combination of proven organ protection, lowered blood glucose, lowered insulin, and weight loss is a powerful incentive for physicians to prescribe these new drugs. Sales have been rising sharply as of 2017, with some analysts predicting that sales could hit $6 billion by 2020.[26]

Alpha-glucosidase inhibitors

Despite the hoopla, the SGLT2 was not actually the first oral hypo-glycemic agent to show proven cardiovascular benefits. Another now largely forgotten drug was previously shown to have similar benefits. Acarbose is an oral diabetes medication first introduced in the United States in 1996. It blocks the enzymes alpha-glucosidase and alpha-amylase, both of which are required for proper digestion of carbohy-drates. Blocking these enzymes prevents complex carbohydrates, which are chains of glucose, from breaking into smaller glucose molecules, thus reducing absorption. Acarbose is essentially the drug equivalent of a low-carbohydrate diet.

The 2003 Study to Prevent Non-Insulin-Dependent Diabetes Mel-litus (STOP-NIDDM)[27] trial showed that acarbose, despite relatively unimpressive lowering of blood glucose, reduced the risk of cardio-vascular events by a remarkable 49 percent and hypertension by 34 percent. In addition to these unprecedented benefits, acarbose also reduced body weight by 1.41 kilograms and waist circumference by 0.79 cm. These results could have been predicted, since blocking absorption of dietary carbohydrates would be expected to lower insulin levels.

At the time of publication, the benefits were ascribed to the blood glucose–lowering effect, and it was expected that more powerful blood glucose–lowering medications would deliver even more impressive benefits. Yet by 2008, the ACCORD, ADVANCE, VADT, and ORIGIN trials had conclusively demonstrated no benefits to blood glucose lowering.

Acarbose succeeded precisely where other medications failed because it reduces both glucotoxicity and insulin toxicity rather than trading one for the other. It is still widely used in China and parts of Asia due to its low cost but is now far less popular in North America because its blood glucose–lowering effect is less powerful and bloating is a bothersome side effect.

Glucagon-like peptide 1 (GLP-1) analogs

Glucagon-like peptide 1 (GLP-1) analogs are diabetic medications that mimic the effect of the incretin hormones. Normally, the incretins secreted by the stomach have several physiological roles when you eat food. They increase the release of insulin but also slow down the motility of the stomach and increase satiety. The DPP-4 inhibitors also enhance incretin levels, but the GLP-1 analogs reach levels that are many times higher than normal.

Incretins increase the insulin response to food, so blood glucose decreases after meals. This transitory rise in insulin is not enough to cause weight gain, but incretins slow the movement of food through the stomach, causing satiety, decreased food intake, and weight loss. It also accounts for the main side effect of nausea and vomiting. The 2016 LEADER trial of the GLP-1 analog Liraglutide showed that nausea occurred four times more often in the drug group than the placebo group.[28] Patients on the medication averaged 2.3 kg weight loss compared to placebo and lowered their A1C by 0.4 percent.

The blood glucose–lowering effect was fairly modest but the cardiovascular benefits were not. Liraglutide could reduce cardiovascular disease and death by approximately 15 percent. While less powerful than the SGLT2 inhibitor class or acarbose, it was still highly significant and promised clinical benefits. Yet again, the glucotoxicity paradigm was proved inadequate to explain what was happening. Clinical benefits only accrue when both glucotoxicity and insulin toxicity are reduced.

A TRADE-OFF, NOT A SOLUTION

STANDARD MEDICATIONS FOR type 2 diabetes represent a trade-off between glucotoxicity and insulin toxicity. Insulin, TZDs, and SUs all increase insulin or its effect to reduce hyperglycemia. The effect of the increased insulin becomes clinically obvious as weight gain. The price of better glucose control has been higher insulin dosage, so there is no net benefit. These medications simply trade lower glucotoxicity for higher insulin toxicity.

Metformin and DPP-4 medications use mechanisms other than raising insulin to lower blood glucose. But they do not lower insulin either, so the result is neither weight gain nor weight loss. Reducing glucotoxicity while keeping insulin neutral produces minimal benefits. Clinically, these medications are weight neutral, but also neutral with regard to cardiovascular risk or benefits.

Acarbose, SGLT2 inhibitors, and GLP-1 analogs all lower glucose but also lower insulin and cause weight loss. Since type 2 diabetes is a disease characterized by elevations in both blood glucose and blood insulin, these medications would be predicted to have the best outcome. And sure enough, that is the case. In a disease of too much insulin, lowering it creates benefits. These three categories of medications could easily be called the good (lowers insulin, body weight, and complications), the bad (neutral), and the ugly (increases insulin, body weight, and complications).

Table 11.1. Oral hypoglycemics in type 2 diabetes: A comparison

	Weight loss	Weight neutral	Weight gain
Drugs	Acarbose SGLT2 inhibitors GLP-1 analogues	Metformin DPP-4 inhibitors	Insulin Sulfonylureas TZDs
Insulin levels	Lowers insulin	Neutral	Raises insulin
Cardiovascular outcomes compared to metformin	Decreases hearts attacks and death	Neutral	Increases heart attacks and death
Verdict?	**GOOD**	**BAD**	**UGLY**

149

The classic oral hypoglycemic agents were exclusively those that were insulin neutral or raised insulin levels. This explains how meta-analyses reviewing all the available literature up to 2016, including twenty randomized controlled trials, could only conclude that "there is no significant evidence of long term efficacy of insulin on any clinical outcome in T2D (type 2 diabetes). However, there is a trend to clinically harmful adverse effects such as hypoglycaemia and weight gain."[29] In other words, insulin treatment, including medications that simulate only the blood glucose–lowering properties of insulin, carries no perceptible benefits and significant risks. Insulin is "significantly more harmful than other active treatments."

A similar review in the *Journal of the American Medical Association* that included all relevant trials up to March 2016 found that none of the drug classes considered, including metformin, SUs, TZDs, and DPP-4 inhibitors, reduced cardiovascular disease or other complications.[30] Importantly, these older medications did not reduce the hyperinsulinemia that is the root problem, or indeed, made it worse. Again, diabetes will continue unless we treat the root cause.

While the scientific evidence is crystal clear, diabetes guidelines are slow to reflect this new reality. Dr. Victor Montori of the Mayo Clinic discovered that 95 percent of published guidelines endorsed the use of diabetes drugs despite their nonexistent benefits.[31] Why would you take medications that have no benefits? Worse, why would you take medications that have no benefits *and* make you fat?

The classic medical treatment, which relies almost exclusively on pharmaceuticals to reduce blood glucose, can therefore best be described as how *not* to treat type 2 diabetes. By contrast, newer agents, which can reduce both blood glucose and insulin levels, show proven benefits to reduce heart and kidney complications of type 2 diabetes. Nevertheless, these medications, while an important step forward, are clearly not the answer; they do not reverse the root cause of type 2 diabetes—our diet. Following a low-fat, calorie-restricted diet and increasing exercise have long been the recommended lifestyle treatment for type 2 diabetes. There is only one problem with this seemingly common sense advice. It doesn't work at all.

12

LOW-CALORIE DIETS
AND EXERCISE:
NOT THE ANSWER

....

N 2015, WHEN Dr. Sarah Hallberg stepped onto the stage at Purdue University to deliver a TEDx talk[1] about reversing diabetes, few in the audience expected to hear what she was about to say: reversing type 2 diabetes starts with *ignoring* the guidelines.

Dr. Hallberg is the medical director of Indiana University's weight loss program, and she argued convincingly that the low-fat diet endorsed by the American Diabetes Association (ADA) and countless medical organizations was almost exactly wrong. These experts were hurting the very patients they hoped to help. Instead, a simple dietary change had the potential to significantly improve diabetes and help weight-loss efforts.

Her lecture soon became an Internet sensation, quickly passing a million views, and she was featured on radio and television and on the front page of the *New York Times Sunday Review.*[2] Her powerful message of hope had struck a chord. And why? *Because it made sense.* So, what exactly are these guidelines that we should ignore?

THE LOW-FAT ERA
. . . .

IN THE EARLY 2000S, the monumental task of recommending an optimal diet for type 2 diabetics was assigned to Dr. Richard Kahn, then the chief medical and scientific officer of the ADA. Like any good scientist, he began by reviewing the available published data. "When you look at the literature, whoa is it weak. It is so weak," he said.[3] But that was not an answer the ADA could give. People demanded dietary advice. So, without any evidence to guide him one way or the other, Dr. Kahn went with the generic advice given to the public at large: to eat a low-fat, high-carbohydrate diet. "It's a diet for all America," he reasoned. Therefore, it should be good for type 2 diabetics, too.

And where did that advice come from? In the U.S., the Senate Select Committee on Nutrition and Human Needs first released its *Dietary Guidelines for Americans* in 1977. Since 1980, the United States Department of Agriculture (USDA) and the Department of Health and Human Services have published a set of dietary guidelines every five years. And in Canada, the federal government has been regularly publishing and updating a food guide since 1942.

The food pyramids published in these guides have been informing our food choices, and doctors' recommendations, ever since. And the foods at the base of the pyramid, the ones to be eaten preferentially, have been grains and other refined carbohydrates. The "bread, rice, cereal, and pasta" group, of which we were supposed to eat six to eleven servings daily, comprise the exact foods that cause the greatest increase in blood glucose. This is also the precise diet that has failed to halt the greatest obesity and type 2 diabetes epidemics the world has ever seen. But let's talk specifically about type 2 diabetes by juxtaposing two incontrovertible facts:

152

1. Type 2 diabetes is characterized by high blood glucose.
2. Refined carbohydrates raise blood glucose levels more than any other foods.

So type 2 diabetics should eat the very foods that raise blood glucose the most? "Illogical" is the only word that comes to mind. Yet, not just the USDA, but also the Diabetes UK, European Association for the Study of Diabetes (EASD), Canadian Diabetes Association, American Heart Association, and National Cholesterol Education Panel recommended fairly similar diets. All of them suggested keeping carbohydrates at a lofty 50 to 60 percent of total calories and dietary fat at less than 30 percent.

The 2008 American Diabetes Association position statement on nutrition advised: "Dietary strategies including reduced calories and reduced intake of dietary fat, can reduce the risk for developing diabetes and are therefore recommended."[4] The logic is hard to follow. Dietary fat does not raise blood glucose. Reducing fat to emphasize carbohydrates, which are known to raise blood glucose, could *protect* against diabetes? How they believed that would work is unknown. It further advised, against all common sense, that "intake of sucrose and sucrose-containing foods by people with diabetes does not need to be restricted." Eating sugar was okay for type 2 diabetics? This could not realistically be expected to lower blood glucose, and the proof came soon enough.

WHY THE LOW FAT ERA BACKFIRED

THE 2012 TREATMENT Options for Type 2 Diabetes in Adolescents and Youths (TODAY) randomized study[5] reduced caloric intake to a miniscule 1200 to 1500 calories per day of a low-fat diet, combined with increased exercise. This followed precisely the recommendations made by the 2008 ADA guidelines. Intensive dietary counseling was provided to ensure compliance in this group of motivated teenagers. Massive effort by both patients and study staff failed to improve blood glucose—and the failure rate was astronomically high. Almost *50 percent* of patients required increased doses and numbers of medications. Whether or not patients followed the recommended lifestyle recommendations *did not matter at all*. Regardless, their diabetes was getting worse, not better. The scariest part of the study was that if these teenagers couldn't do it, what hope did middle-aged or elderly adults have?

This classic "Eat Less, Move More" strategy failed yet again. But the fact that this diet would not work should have been fairly obvious from the beginning. Reducing dietary fat means increasing dietary carbohydrates, since it is difficult to eat protein alone. In the Westernized world, these carbohydrates were not leafy greens but the refined grains and sugars that increase blood glucose and insulin maximally.

What was certainly behind the recommendation of a low-fat diet was the belief that lowering dietary fat could protect against heart disease and stroke. The most common cause of death in type 2 diabetes is cardiovascular disease, which had been falsely attributed to dietary fat. It must surely have been predicted that diabetes would worsen on this low-fat but high-carbohydrate regimen, but presumably the benefits were felt to be worth this risk. Upon closer inspection, these illusory benefits burst like a ripe abscess.

By 1997, the Nurses' Health Study (see chapter 4), a massive observational study from Harvard University, found no relationship between dietary fat or dietary cholesterol and heart disease.[6] The final nail in the coffin was the 2006 Women's Health Initiative (also in chapter 4).[7] Almost 50,000 women followed this low-fat, calorie-reduced diet for more than eight years,[8] yet the rates of heart disease and stroke did not improve whatsoever. And despite good compliance with years of calorie restriction, on average women lost less than a quarter of a pound.

There were absolutely no tangible benefits to long-term compliance with a low-fat diet.[9] Other studies quickly reached the same conclusions. Despite forty years of research trying to link dietary fat, dietary cholesterol, and heart disease, not a single shred of evidence could be found.[10]

In diabetic patients, the story was the same. The Action for Health in Diabetes (LookAHEAD) clinical trial studied more than 5000 obese patients with type 2 diabetes at sixteen sites across the U.S. The researchers compared a control group receiving standard diabetes intervention with a second group that ate only 1200 to 1800 calories per day, less than 30 percent of them from fat, and did 175 minutes per week of moderate-intensity physical activity.[11] This was the recommended "intensive lifestyle intervention" of every diabetes association in the world. Would it reduce heart disease as promised?

In a word, no. In 2012, the trial was stopped early after 9.6 years of high hopes. The data indicated there was no chance patients would show cardiovascular benefits and continuing the study was futile. Researchers threw in the towel. The low-fat, calorie-reduced diet had failed yet again.

All the scientific evidence has consistently refuted the dearly held belief that reducing dietary fat would lead to weight loss and reduce heart disease.[12] Finally, the 2015 *Dietary Guidelines for Americans* (the most recent) have removed the limits on dietary fat intake to reflect this new understanding, recognizing that there are a number of healthy fats, such as those found in olive oil, nuts, and avocados. The low-fat, calorie-reduced diet was a bust.

THE EXERCISE APPROACH

LIFESTYLE INTERVENTIONS, TYPICALLY a combination of diet and exercise, are a universally acknowledged mainstay of type 2 diabetes treatments. These two stalwarts are often portrayed as equally beneficial, and why not?

Exercise improves weight-loss efforts, although its effects are much more modest than most assume. Nevertheless, physical inactivity is an independent risk factor for more than twenty-five chronic diseases, including type 2 diabetes and cardiovascular disease.[13] Low levels of physical activity in obese subjects are a better predictor of death than cholesterol levels, smoking status, or blood pressure.[14]

And the benefits of exercise extend far beyond simple weight loss. Exercise programs improve strength and balance, blood pressure, cholesterol, blood glucose, and insulin sensitivity, without involving medications and their potential side effects. Trained athletes have consistently lower insulin levels, and these benefits can be maintained for

155

life, as demonstrated by many studies on older athletes. These seem like good returns for a low-cost investment.

Yet results of both aerobic and resistance exercise studies in type 2 diabetes are varied.[15,16] Meta-analyses show that exercise may significantly reduce A1C, without a change in body mass. This finding suggests that exercise does not need to reduce body weight to have benefits, which echoes clinical experience with patients. However, the corollary is that exercise programs have minimal effect for weight loss.

With all the proven benefits of exercise, it may surprise you to learn that I think this is *not* useful information. Why not? *Because everybody already knows this.* The benefits of exercise have been extolled relentlessly for the past forty years. I have yet to meet a single person who has not already understood that exercise might help type 2 diabetes and heart disease. If people already know its importance, what is the point of telling them again?

The main problem has always been noncompliance. Many real issues may deter someone from embarking on an exercise program: obesity itself, joint pain, neuropathy, peripheral vascular disease, back pain, and heart disease may all combine to make exercise difficult or even unsafe. Overall, however, I suspect the biggest issue is lack of visible results. The benefits are greatly overhyped and exercise doesn't work nearly as well as advertised. Weight loss is often minimal. This lack of results despite great effort is demoralizing.

THE DISAPPOINTING IMPACT OF EXERCISE

CONCEPTUALLY, EXERCISE SEEMS like an ideal way to burn off the excess ingested calories of glucose. Standard recommendations are to exercise thirty minutes per day, five days per week, for a total of 150 minutes per week. At a modest pace, the result is an extra energy expenditure of 150 to 200 kcal per day, or 700 to 1000 kcal per week. These amounts pale in comparison to a total energy intake of 14,000 calories per week.

In studies, all exercise programs produce substantially fewer benefits than expected. There are two main reasons: First, exercise is known to stimulate appetite. This tendency to eat more after exercise reduces expected weight loss. Second, a formal exercise program tends to decrease non-exercise activity. For example, if you have been doing hard physical labor all day, you are unlikely to come home and run 10 kilometers for fun. On the other hand, if you've been sitting in front of the computer all day, that 10-kilometer run might sound pretty good. These compensation effects are a well-described phenomenon in exercise studies. As you increase exercise intensity or duration, you may find that you eat more or do fewer other non-exercise activities. These compensations directly reduce the beneficial effects of the exercise program.

In the end, the main problem is that type 2 diabetes *is not caused by lack of exercise*. The underlying problem is excessive dietary glucose and fructose causing hyperinsulinemia. Exercise can only improve insulin resistance of the muscles. It does not improve insulin resistance in the liver at all. The fatty liver is the key to developing type 2 diabetes, and you cannot exercise your liver to health. Reversing type 2 diabetes depends upon treating the root cause of the disease, which is dietary.

Imagine that you turn on your bathroom faucet full blast. The sink starts to fill quickly, as the drain is small. Widening the drain slightly is not the solution because it does not address the underlying problem. The obvious solution is to turn off the faucet. In type 2 diabetes, a diet full of refined carbohydrates and sugars is filling our bodies quickly with glucose and fructose. Widening the drain by exercising is minimally effective. The obvious solution is to turn off the faucet. And that leads us to the next section, how to effectively treat type 2 diabetes.

ELENA

Elena, 63, was diagnosed with type 2 diabetes three years before I met her. She also had a history of high blood pressure, high cholesterol, and obesity—the classic manifestations of metabolic syndrome—and evidence of fatty liver damage. She was taking metformin for diabetes as well as medications to lower her blood pressure and cholesterol. Her A1C was 6.2%.

When Elena joined the IDM program, we discussed low-carbohydrate, healthy-fat diets and she began a fasting regimen of 36 hours, three times per week. Having long been told to eat frequent small meals throughout the day, fasting required a new mindset. Within two weeks of starting the program, however, she was able to stop taking metformin. A year after she began, she also stopped taking hypertension medication, as her blood pressure had normalized. At our last meeting, her A1C was 5.2%, which is well within the normal range.

Today, Elena is considered nondiabetic. The blood markers that indicate liver damage have completely normalized, meaning she no longer suffers from the fatty liver that causes chronic liver damage. Furthermore, she has dropped 60 pounds, lost 24 cm off her waist, and completely reversed her metabolic syndrome.

RICHARD

Richard, 76, was diagnosed with type 2 diabetes about a decade ago. In addition, he had high blood pressure, stroke, peripheral vascular disease, an irregular heartbeat (atrial fibrillation), and chronic kidney disease. Six years later he started on insulin (36 units daily), in addition to two oral hypoglycemics, yet his A1C remained elevated at 8.4%.

I met Richard just after he started taking insulin. Following the IDM program, he began a low-carbohydrate, healthy-fat diet and a 24-hour fast three days per week. Within a month he was off insulin, and after six months he was completely off all his oral medications, as well. His urine albumin-to-creatinine ratio, a measure of diabetic kidney damage, dropped by two-thirds; he lost 13 pounds; and his waist size shrank by 12 cm. Today, Richard's A1C is 5.4% without medications, which classifies him as nondiabetic.

PART
FIVE

How to Effectively
Treat Type 2 Diabetes

LESSONS FROM
BARIATRIC SURGERY

....

T 203 KILOGRAMS (448 pounds), Adrian was morbidly obese
and suffered from type 2 diabetes. Medically unfit to work due to
all his associated illnesses, he lost his job in 2014. He eventually
chose to undertake weight-loss surgery, also called bariatric surgery,
and within five weeks his diabetes had completely disappeared.[1] Interestingly, this story of type 2 diabetes reversal is not the exception but a
general rule after surgery.

How often have we heard type 2 diabetes called a chronic and progressive disease? This idea has only become accepted as if it were fact
because we have spent decades treating the symptom (hyperglycemia)
rather than the cause. Bariatric surgery proves that this notion is simply mistaken: type 2 diabetes is a reversible and preventable disease.
When we treat the cause (hyperinsulinemia), we can reverse diabetes.
Remember Dr. Hallberg's advice in chapter 12: ignore the guidelines.
What does bariatrics teach us about type 2 diabetes? Quite a lot, it
turns out.

EARLY ATTEMPTS AT WEIGHT-LOSS SURGERY

THE EARLIEST ATTEMPT to surgically cure obesity was to simply wire the jaws shut. The logic is obvious, if not very imaginative. This restrictive treatment, though, was ultimately unsuccessful. Patients could still drink fluids, and enough high-calorie sugary drinks derailed weight loss. The severe side effects were the limiting factor. Dental infections and vomiting were insurmountable problems that often progressed over time. More often than not, these intolerable problems led to reversing the surgery.[2]

In 1925, the *Lancet* noted that partial removal of the stomach for peptic ulcer disease often caused weight loss and complete resolution of sugar in the urine, now called diabetes.[3] The smaller stomach volume effectively reduced the amount a person could eat. Similar reports followed sporadically in the 1950s and 1960s. This was an interesting finding, but the results often did not endure. Over time, the smaller stomach could expand and patients could eat normally. Weight would rebound, and with it, type 2 diabetes.

Jejunocolic bypass surgery

The modern age of bariatric surgery began in 1963 with the observation that removal of the small bowel, which absorbs most of the ingested nutrients, caused significant weight loss. This led to the development of the jejunocolic bypass operation, in which bypassing the small bowel reroutes food from the stomach directly to the colon. Success! Patients lost significant amounts of weight using this malabsorptive approach.

But the side effects became immediately obvious. Bypassing the small bowel did not allow the food to undergo the normal digestive process. This was the point: if the food passed right through, it could not hang around long enough to be absorbed and eventually stored as body fat. Instead, this food energy was immediately excreted in the stool. However, this rapid passage also meant essential food nutrients were not absorbed properly or at all. Patients developed night blindness from vitamin A deficiency, and osteoporosis from vitamin D deficiency. Other common problems included severe diarrhea and bacterial overgrowth, liver failure, and kidney stones. The continual diarrhea from the malabsorbed fat led to anal excoriations and hemorrhoids. No fun. This procedure, too, was soon abandoned.

Jejunoileal bypass

These complications forced the switch to the less-intensive jejunoileal bypass, in which most, but not all, of the small bowel is bypassed by rerouting food from the stomach directly to a very short section of the small bowel. Although absorption improved slightly, the complications were still unacceptable, rendering this surgery a historical footnote. However, this incremental improvement allowed others to build upon these initial experiences.

In 1967, the seed of modern bariatric surgical procedures was planted with the use of restrictive and malabsorptive components combined. This approach physically limited the intake of food by removing most of the stomach, and also reduced the absorption of whatever food made it through. In addition to the partial bypass of the small bowel, part of the stomach was removed. With the basic idea in place, further refinements were added over time.

WEIGHT-LOSS SURGERY TODAY

COMPARED TO THE number of obese people in the United States, the number of bariatric surgeries remains very small. In 2015, approximately 200,000 weight-loss surgeries were performed in the United States.[4] Outside the U.S., this procedure is performed even less often, though there are few reliable statistics.

165

Roux-En-Y gastric bypass

The standard form of bariatric surgery today is Roux-En-Y gastric bypass, which takes its name from the creation of a blind loop of the small bowel that makes a Y shape of the small intestines. Most of the healthy stomach is removed until the only portion remaining is approximately the size of a walnut, which severely restricts food intake. By itself, this procedure serves as only a short-term solution, so the second step of the surgery involves rerouting the small intestine to prevent the absorption of most, but not all, of the ingested food.

This combined restrictive and malabsorptive procedure makes the Roux-En-Y bypass the current heavyweight champion of bariatric surgeries, with the best weight loss but also the most complications. This surgery has "Go big or go home" tattooed on its massive bicep. In addition to the usual risks of bleeding and infection common to all surgeries, deficiencies of all nutrients, including proteins, vitamins, and minerals, can lead to lifelong malnutrition after the bypass. Gastric dumping syndrome, caused when food moves too quickly (is dumped) from the surgically altered stomach to the small intestines, can cause nausea, diarrhea, and facial flushing after meals. Strictures (abnormal narrowings) due to scar tissue can occur at the surgical site and block the passage to the stomach.

The Roux-En-Y surgery is often reserved for severe cases of obesity, typically patients with a body mass index greater than 40. The side effects, however, have led to the development of milder forms of bariatric surgery that can also produce spectacular results without the complexity or complications of the Roux-En-Y.

The sleeve gastrectomy

The sleeve gastrectomy simply removes a large portion of the healthy stomach without altering the intestines, making it a purely restrictive form of weight-loss surgery. It dramatically reduces the stomach's capacity for holding food. More than a thimbleful of food causes severe gastric distention, ballooning of the miniature stomach, and persistent nausea and vomiting. Over time, the remaining stomach stretches until it becomes possible to eat small meals.

Since this procedure may be done laparoscopically—through a series of small incisions—there tend to be fewer acute surgical complications

166

such as bleeding and infection. Although gastric dumping syndrome is rare after this procedure, strictures are common. More importantly, perhaps, compared to the Roux-En-Y surgery, it leads to less weight loss and less durable results.

The gastric "lap" band

An even simpler surgery is the surgically implanted gastric "lap" band that wraps around the stomach. Like cinching a tight belt, the lap band restricts food from entering the stomach. No part of the healthy stomach is removed, and the lap band can be gradually tightened or loosened as needed. Because of its relative simplicity, this procedure has the fewest complications and can be used by anybody for weight loss. The main problem is that weight is often regained over time. One surgeon, a friend, remarked that the most common lap band surgery these days is its removal.

Figure 13.1. Gastric lap banding

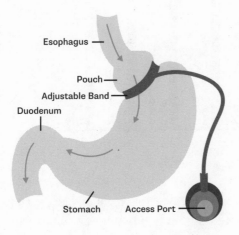

Esophagus

Pouch

Adjustable Band

Duodenum

Stomach   Access Port

In the short term, all types of bariatric surgery have been proved effective for weight loss and diabetes. Longer-term studies show varied effectiveness,[5] depending upon the type of surgery. However, I do not wish to praise or condemn any of these surgeries. As with everything else in medicine, they have their place. My main question is: what happens to type 2 diabetes after bariatric surgery? What does bariatric surgery teach us?

WHY BARIATRIC SURGERY WORKS

IN VIRTUALLY ALL cases, type 2 diabetes completely disappears after bariatric surgery. Type 2 diabetes is entirely reversible, even in a 500-pound patient with a twenty-year duration of disease. It is not only reversible, but *rapidly* reversible. In a matter of weeks, the diabetes disappears. Yes, it truly just goes away.

Figure 13.2. Surgery cures diabetes[6]

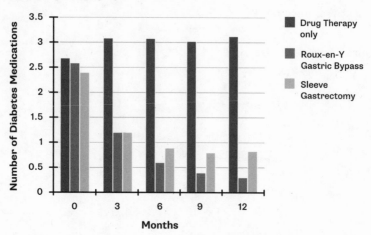

A 2012 trial called Surgical Treatment and Medications Potentially Eradicate Diabetes Efficiently (STAMPEDE)[7] compared the effects of gastric bypass surgery with intensive medical therapy (drug treatments) on obese type 2 diabetics with very high blood glucose levels. Surgical patients did amazingly well. Within three months, most patients stopped taking all their diabetic medications because their blood glucose had normalized, often long before they noticed substantial weight loss. Technically, these patients no longer had diabetes. In other words, type 2 diabetes is reversible—even curable.

By contrast, the patients in the intensive medical therapy group experienced no improvement in their disease over time. They continued to require ever-increasing doses of medications for type 2 diabetes.

Super-obese adolescents (with an average body mass index of 53) undergoing bariatric surgery have enjoyed the same success,[8] maintaining a ninety-pound weight loss over three years. High blood pressure resolved in 74 percent of patients, and abnormal lipids in 66 percent of them. And type 2 diabetes? Glad you asked. A stunning 95 *percent* of type 2 diabetes was reversed: by trial's end, these patients had a median A1C of only 5.3 percent without medications. Once again, this would classify these patients as nondiabetic.

That surgery can reverse type 2 diabetes has been known since 1992,[9] when a study found that patients who had undergone bariatric surgery achieved normal blood glucose within two months and maintained it for ten years. The benefits extended far beyond their body weight. Many of their metabolic abnormalities normalized as well. Sky-high insulin levels plummeted to normal levels. Blood glucose dropped in half. Fasting insulin, a marker of insulin resistance, dropped 73 percent.

What lesson can be learned from this? The problem was *not* that the disease was chronic and progressive. The problem was that our treatment didn't really work. We had seen the great enemy, and it was ourselves.

The startling success of bariatric surgery led to a 2016 joint statement supported by forty-five diabetes organizations—including such influential groups as the American Diabetes Association, the International Diabetes Federation, and Diabetes UK—that surgery be recommended as a first-line treatment option for patients with type 2 diabetes and a body mass index greater than 40, regardless of other lifestyle interventions.[10] At a body mass index between 35 and 40, they suggested, surgery should be considered only if other lifestyle options

169

failed. With this endorsement, these groups have tacitly admitted that standard medications and lifestyle treatments (low-fat, low-calorie diets) have failed to effectively treat this disease.

WHY SURGERY IS NOT USUALLY THE RIGHT SOLUTION

DESPITE THE SUCCESS of all these surgeries, I don't generally recommend them for a variety of reasons. Surgery carries a heavy price, both financially and physiologically, due to many surgical complications. Most importantly, though, *we can derive all these amazing benefits without surgery.* We only need to understand why surgery succeeds where other approaches fail, and how we can duplicate its results.

Many theories have tried to explain this. The foregut hypothesis suggested that removing part of the healthy stomach is responsible for the myriad of benefits. The stomach secretes many hormones, including incretins, peptide YY, and ghrelin. Removing the stomach reduces all of these hormones, and perhaps others not yet identified. However, it soon became obvious that this explanation cannot possibly be correct.

The less-invasive gastric banding does not remove any part of the stomach, but reverses type 2 diabetes as effectively as the Roux-En-Y procedure in the short term. Indeed, the different bariatric procedures do not differ substantially in their ability to reduce insulin resistance, despite the wide variation in stomach removal or rerouting of the small intestines. The only variable that matters is how much weight is lost.

The foregut hypothesis also failed to explain why type 2 diabetes often recurs years later, since the stomach does not regenerate the ability to secrete these hormones. This reasoning proves what should have been a rather obvious point: that removing the healthy stomach doesn't truly have any benefits.

The "fat mass" hypothesis suggests that the loss of the fat tissue leads to the beneficial effects. Adipocytes actively secrete many different hormones, and perhaps one or several of these is the problem. For

170

example, adipocytes convert testosterone into estrogen, leading to the familiar phenomenon of "man boobs" in obesity. So adipocytes are not metabolically inert, but active hormonal players. This thinking presents two problems: First, type 2 diabetes disappears within weeks of surgery, long before any substantial loss of fatty mass. Second, liposuction removes fat but fails to provide any metabolic benefit. It does not significantly improve blood glucose readings or any measurable metabolic markers. It offers only cosmetic benefits.[11]

There is no real magic here. The mechanism of benefit is the simplest and most obvious. All bariatric surgeries are effective because they create *a sudden, severe caloric reduction*. The simplest explanation is often the correct one.

Remember that insulin resistance is an overflow phenomenon. Our liver cells are jammed full of sugar and fat, like an overinflated balloon. Insulin signals the cell to open up the gates to allow glucose inside. The overflowing liver cells turn away the glucose, leaving it in the blood and triggering the phenomenon known as insulin resistance. To decompress the congested liver, newly created fat is exported to other organs, clogging up the pancreas and leading to lowered insulin secretion.

With sudden, severe caloric restriction, our body depletes liver glycogen stores in about twenty-four hours. Once that's gone, we are forced to burn fat for energy. The body burns the fat from the liver and other organs preferentially, because it is more accessible than the fat stored in the adipocytes.

Recall that this fat, contained within and around the abdominal organs, causes metabolic syndrome. Therefore, removing this ectopic, visceral fat reverses type 2 diabetes long before any substantial reduction in overall fat mass becomes apparent. Diabetes reverses within weeks of surgery, even though patients are still hundreds of pounds overweight.

Removing fat from the organs leads to rapid metabolic improvement. Removing excess fat from the pancreas resolves beta cell dysfunction. As insulin secretion returns to normal, blood glucose begins to drop. Removing the excess fat from the liver, like deflating that overinflated balloon, reverses insulin resistance. The dual defects of type 2 diabetes resolve.

What these surgical success stories show conclusively is that type 2 diabetes *is a fully reversible disease.* We have been led to believe that type 2 diabetes progresses inevitably, like age. But this belief is simply not true. Let's juxtapose two facts:

- Type 2 diabetes is a largely reversible disease.
- With the standard treatments of low-calorie, reduced-fat diets and medications (including insulin), type 2 diabetes progresses.

The only logical conclusion here, as bizarre as it may sound, is that most cases of type 2 diabetes are being treated *incorrectly.* That is why type 2 diabetes has become an epidemic. The problem is not the disease but our treatment and understanding of it.

The reason that sudden, severe caloric restriction reverses type 2 diabetes is that it forces the body to burn the fat stored within the bloated liver and pancreas cells. The body simply burns off the excess sugar and fat that causes the type 2 diabetes and the disease goes into remission. So is there another way to burn off all that ectopic fat without the cost and complications of surgery? As it happens, there is. As Dr. Sarah Hallberg and Dr. Osama Hamdy wrote in the *New York Times,* "Before you spend $26,000 on weight loss surgery, do this."[12] What is the solution they're talking about? Simple. A low-carbohydrate diet.

CARBOHYDRATE-REDUCED
DIETS

....

If I had a flood in my house…
I would not spend day after day, week after week, &
year after year buying buckets, mops and towels. I would not be
inventing different types of buckets and more expensive
mops or drainage systems to ensure the water drained away quickly.
I would find the source of the water and turn it off!

DR. VERNER WHEELOCK

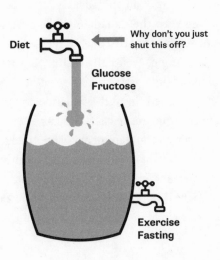

I N 2015, NEWSPAPERS reported that a three-year-old Texan girl had become the world's youngest person to develop type 2 diabetes.[1] Yes, three years old. At birth, she weighed 3.2 kg (7 pounds). At three-and-a-half years old, she weighed 35 kg (77 pounds) and presented to the hospital with the classic symptoms of diabetes: frequent urination and thirst.

Given her age, medical staff naturally assumed she had type 1 diabetes, the so-called early onset or juvenile diabetes. However, her obesity suggested type 2 diabetes, and further testing confirmed it. There was no family history of diabetes. Instead the problem was her diet, which consisted mostly of candy, sugary drinks, and fast food. The toddler was initially placed on medications. But with the proper diet, she lost 25 percent of her original weight and was able to stop taking all her medications as her blood glucose levels returned to normal. Two years later, this little girl's diabetes was cured.

Here's another heart-warming story. My friend Betsy (not her real name) was a twenty-seven-year-old medical researcher in a local academic hospital. At her yearly checkup, she was overweight but otherwise felt well. She was shocked to learn that screening blood tests revealed a hemoglobin A1C of 10.4, which meant she had severe type 2 diabetes. Alarmed, her physician immediately prescribed three different medications in line with the Canadian Diabetes Association guidelines. Betsy was further warned that she would likely need medications for the rest of her life and, eventually, insulin. She heard that type 2 diabetes is chronic and progressive, a disease without hope of a cure.

Horrified, Betsy rejected this dire prediction and took none of the medications. She did some research, started a very low-carbohydrate diet called a ketogenic diet, and immediately noticed a difference. Her weight dropped. Her waist size shrank. Three months later, her A1C level was only 5.5 percent without any medications at all. She looked and felt great. By definition, she no longer had type 2 diabetes. Again, Betsy's diabetes was cured. So much for a chronic and progressive disease!

In both cases, dietary changes addressed the root cause and reversed the diabetes. That's no surprise. All diabetes associations throughout the world recommend starting treatment with diet and lifestyle changes before prescribing medication. But what's the best diet to follow for type 2 diabetes? Unfortunately, that's a more difficult question.

THE FAILURE OF THE LOW-FAT DIET

THE WORLD HEALTH Organization released its first *Global Report on Diabetes* in 2016 but it only provides vague, general dietary guidelines for treatment.[2] It says that added sugars should be reduced to less than 10 percent of total calories but mentions nothing about optimal macronutrient composition. There is no guidance to follow a low- or high-carbohydrate, low- or high-fat, low- or high-protein diet. Similarly, the American Diabetes Association 2016 standards of care document, *Diabetes Care,*[3] declined to recommend any particular diet. Both of these organizations have quietly backed away from the ineffective low-fat, calorie-restriction dietary advice they had promoted for forty years, tacitly acknowledging its futility.

Fatty but delicious foods such as butter, full-fat cheese, and cream were said to "clog arteries" and cause heart disease, so the *Dietary Guidelines for Americans* in 1977 recommended that people eat 50 to 60 percent of their total daily calories as carbohydrates, in order to lower dietary fat. Even as recently as 2008, the American Diabetes Association position paper recommended a minimum daily carbohydrate intake of 130 grams.[4] In North America, these carbohydrates tend to be highly refined wheat and corn products such as sugar, bread, and pasta.

In 1999, at the height of the low-fat mania, the landmark Lyon Diet Heart Study sent shockwaves through the medical community.[5] Patients who had suffered heart attacks were randomly assigned to the American Heart Association's low-fat diet or the high-fat Mediterranean diet, which was full of olive oil, nuts, and avocados. The results were almost unbelievable. The Mediterranean diet reduced heart disease and death by a jaw-dropping 75 percent. It should hardly have come as a surprise, as it confirmed what used to be called the French paradox.

In the 1980s and 1990s, people in France were eating saturated fat like it was going out of style, yet their death rate from cardiovascular disease was less than half what it was in the U.S. If saturated fat clogged arteries and led inexorably to heart disease, then how could the French possibly eat more fat and have less heart disease? The answer, in hindsight, is pretty obvious. Eating saturated fat does *not* lead to cardiovascular disease.[6]

The cardiovascular benefits of the relatively high-fat Mediterranean diet have since been replicated many times. Most recently, the 2013 PREDIMED study confirmed that patients on the Mediterranean diet reduced their rate of heart disease and death.[7] Further comparison of different dietary habits in the countries of Europe in 2012 shows that higher saturated fat intake is associated with *less* heart disease.[8] A 2009 meta-analysis[9] demonstrated that saturated fat had no correlation to heart disease and offers slight protection against stroke. In Japan, this protection against stroke has also been noted.[10] Slowly but steadily, the realization that diets high in natural fats are intrinsically healthy is gaining ground.

Figure 14.1. Higher dietary fat = lower risk of stroke and heart attack[11]

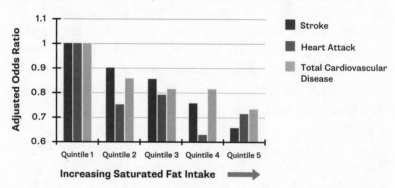

WHY TO EAT HEALTHY FAT
....

THE NUTRITIONAL LANDSCAPE began to change in the mid-2000s, as foods high in monounsaturated fats began to be recommended for heart health. Avocados, once regarded as dangerous due to their high fat content, are now highly valued as a healthy superfood. Similarly, eating more nuts is routinely linked to better health outcomes. Daily nut consumption is associated with a 35 percent decreased risk of heart attack.[12]

Fatty cold-water fish, which are rich in omega-3 oil, are also considered extremely protective against heart disease. Northern communities where native people have eaten a traditional diet full of whale and seal blubber as well as fatty fish have had virtually no cardiovascular disease or type 2 diabetes.[13] The town of Upernavik, Greenland, for example, reported only a single case of type 2 diabetes between 1950 and 1974; in comparison, about 13 percent of Americans currently suffer from this disease.

High blood levels of trans-palmitoleic acid from full-fat dairy are associated with a 60 percent reduction in the incidence of type 2 diabetes. It also improves HDL triglyceride levels and lowers markers of inflammation, such as high-sensitivity C-reactive protein.[14] Egg yolks, once reviled as being high in cholesterol, have been vindicated. Studies now conclude that eating eggs, even daily, does *not* raise the risk of heart disease.[15] In fact, consuming lots of eggs reduces the risk of diabetes by 42 percent.[16]

Why is fat useful in preventing and treating type 2 diabetes? Remember that of the three macronutrients, dietary fat stimulates insulin the least. Pure fats, such as butter and olive oil, stimulate almost no insulin release. Therefore, replacing refined carbohydrates with natural fats is a simple, natural method of reducing insulin.[17]

WHY TO REDUCE REFINED CARBOHYDRATES

IN 2001, IN a critical review of dietary fat and cardiovascular disease, Dr. Walter Willett of Harvard's School of Public Health noted that, "It is now increasingly recognized that the low-fat campaign has been based on little scientific evidence and may have caused unintended health consequences."[18] Furthermore, as shown by Figure 14.2 from the Nurses' Health Study, a very large, long-term observational study from Harvard University, he found a clear correlation between high glycemic load in the diet and the risk of heart disease.[19]

Sugar and refined carbohydrates have a high glycemic load, which raises blood glucose and the risk of type 2 diabetes. This, in turn, significantly increases the risk of heart disease.

Figure 14.2. Higher glycemic load = higher risk of heart disease[20]

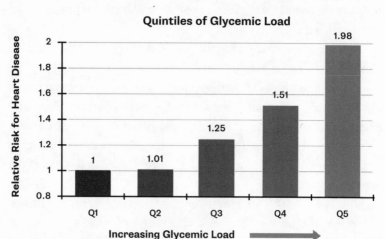

A comprehensive 2013 review concluded that certain diets provide superior glycemic control.[21] Specifically, four were found beneficial: the low-carbohydrate diet, low glycemic-index diet, Mediterranean diet, and high-protein diet. All four diets share a common trait: they reduce dietary carbohydrates to varying degrees. Low-carbohydrate diets have proven more effective at reducing body weight, waist size, and blood glucose.[22]

Figure 14.3. U.S. Macronutrient Consumption 1965–2011[23]

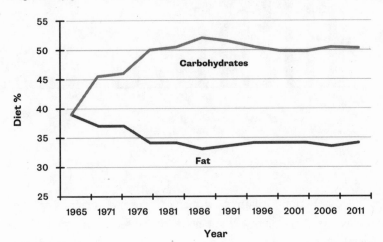

Data from the National Health and Nutrition Examination Survey (NHANES) show that between 1965 and 2000, as the twin epidemics of obesity and type 2 diabetes unfolded, Americans primarily ate more carbohydrates and less dietary fat as a percentage of diet, just as the dietary guidelines recommended.[24]

Refined grains and sugars are the main sources of carbohydrates, and any low-carbohydrate diet should restrict these. Yet we need to make a further distinction between unrefined carbohydrates, such as potatoes and fruit, and refined carbohydrates, such as added sugars and flour, because the higher the intake of refined carbohydrates, the higher the risk of diabetes.[25] The reason is that refined carbohydrates increase blood glucose higher and faster than unrefined ones. This effect becomes obvious when looking at glycemic load. Unrefined foods score low on the scale despite having similar amounts of dietary carbohydrates.

179

Figure 14.4. Glycemic load of various carbohydrates[26]

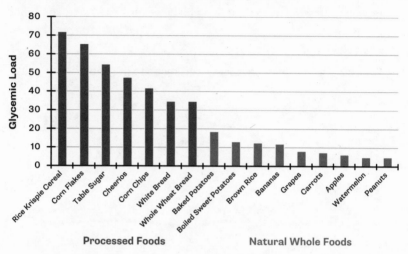

This distinction explains how many traditional societies can eat carbohydrate-based diets without evidence of disease. For example, the Tukisenta, a highland tribe of New Guinea, derive 94.6 percent of their energy intake as whole, unprocessed carbohydrates; and the Okinawans, a group living on a small island in southern Japan, eat a traditional diet that is almost 85 percent starch. Both groups eat mostly sweet potatoes. With virtually no sugar or refined grains such as flour,[27] type 2 diabetes is almost non-existent. The native diet of Kitava, a small island off New Guinea, consists of 69 percent carbohydrates, mostly tubers (sweet potato, cassava, and yam), coconut, and fruit, but their average insulin level is lower than 90 percent of Swedes.[28]

In other words, higher carbohydrate intake alone does not necessarily lead to higher insulin levels. Refining and processing plays a leading role in enhancing the insulin effect. Removing the natural fiber, fat, and proteins in foods leaves pure concentrated carbohydrates, a form not found naturally. Further grinding of these carbohydrates into a fine powder (such as flour) increases the speed of digestion, which results in higher blood glucose spikes. At the same time, we tend to eat more refined carbohydrates because the satiating effect of the protein, fiber, and fat have been lost. Fructose plays a dominant role in the development of fatty liver, insulin resistance, and hyperinsulinemia, and traditional societies eat little or no added sugar.

The essential defect of type 2 diabetes is hyperinsulinemia, which may or may not be the result of too many carbohydrates. Reversing or preventing type 2 diabetes means lowering insulin, and even diets high in carbohydrates may do that. However, avoiding sugar and refined carbohydrates remains the cornerstone of success. Studies prove that a reduced-carbohydrate, higher-fat Mediterranean diet using olive oil reduces the need for medication by a stunning 59 percent.[29] By recognizing the potential benefits of eating natural fats and reducing the amount of added sugars and processed, refined carbohydrates, we are on our way to reducing and reversing type 2 diabetes.

GET RID OF SUGAR—GET RID OF DIABETES

WE KNOW THAT the very essence of type 2 diabetes is too much sugar in the body, not just in the blood. Once we understand this basic paradigm, the solution is immediately obvious. If the problem is too much sugar (glucose and fructose), two treatments will work. And luckily, neither involves surgery or medications:

1. Stop putting sugar in (low-carbohydrate diets, intermittent fasting).
2. Burn remaining sugar off (intermittent fasting).

In short, a natural, drug-free solution to type 2 diabetes now lies within our grasp.

Diets that eliminate sugar short-circuit the vicious cycle of too much glucose leading to insulin resistance, insulin toxicity, and disease. Remember, eating triggers insulin, but different macronutrients require different amounts of insulin. Fat breaks down into fatty acids, which don't need insulin to properly metabolize. Protein breaks down into amino acids, which need a little insulin to allow them to be processed by the liver. Carbohydrates are the big insulin hogs. They break

181

down into glucose, which requires insulin to get into the cells. Fructose, found in sugar and high-fructose corn syrup, directly causes insulin resistance, which leads back to hyperinsulinemia. Due to its unique metabolic pathway, fructose is many times more likely to cause insulin resistance than glucose.

There are many reasons to recommend a diet low in carbohydrates for type 2 diabetes.[30] Don't just take my word for it; low-carbohydrate diets have been practiced in various forms for centuries, dating back to the writings of William Banting in 1863.[31] Doctors all over the world are slowly recognizing the profound power of dietary change to influence the treatment of diabetes.

I asked Dr. David Unwin, the winner of the United Kingdom's prestigious National Health Service Innovator of the Year Award in 2016, to contribute a section to this book. He emailed me the following description of his experience working as a family doctor in Northern England:

> I had an emergency call from the lab about a "sky-high" blood glucose result. I rushed over to [my patient's] house and found her just about to have lunch, spoon in hand over two large bowls, one of vanilla ice cream and the second of rice pudding with a packet of chocolate buttons. I gave her a stark choice: either eat less sugar or start lifelong insulin. Within a week of choosing a better diet, her blood sugar settled into a normal range. Her case looks rather obvious, but I wonder if our choices are always as apparent?
>
> For the first two-thirds of my career as a doctor, I was ignorant of the truly amazing power of simply severely cutting back on sugar. It was, in truth, my patients that taught me this crucial lesson. One decided to give up dietary sugar and quickly proceeded to lose 23 kg. She normalised her blood glucose and blood pressure, and no longer required four different "lifelong" medications. Years later, now aged 70, she is healthy, strong, and rides everywhere on her bicycle. Strange, I thought. I had been telling everybody about the chronic, progressive nature of diabetes as I ramped up the medications.

Another patient just stopped her diabetes medication. Worried, I called her. She had lost so much weight, and looked so young that I thought it was the wrong patient. She started eating a low-carbohydrate diet where not just sugar but all sources of glucose are greatly reduced. Blood tests confirmed her diabetes was into full remission.

A week later, an article in the *British Medical Journal* caught my eye. Bread raised blood glucose more than table sugar. Disbelieving, I found to my utter amazement—it's a fact! Starchy foods like bread, cereals, rice, or potato are "concentrated" sugar, digested into huge amounts of glucose. The Glycaemic Index predicts how various carbohydrate-containing foods will affect blood glucose. Changing the scale into equivalents of teaspoons of sugar led to some surprising results. (Note: This is for illustrative purposes only. Foods listed are not identical to sugar since sugar contains both fructose and glucose.)

Figure 14.5. How foods affect blood glucose: A comparison[32]

Food Item	G Index	Serve size (g)	How does each food affect blood glucose compared with one 4g teaspoon of table sugar?
Boiled rice	69	150	10.1
Boiled potato	96	150	9.1
French fries	64	150	7.5
Spaghetti, boiled	39	180	6.6
Sweet corn, boiled	60	80	4.0
Frozen peas, boiled	51	80	1.3
Banana	62	120	5.7
Apple	39	120	2.3
Wholemeal, small slice	74	30	3.0
Broccoli	54	80	0.2
Eggs	0	60	0

Armed with this new knowledge, I started to treat all motivated diabetic patients in my practice with a low-carbohydrate diet. So far after four years, 160 patients have tried it, with amazing results:

- Average weight loss of 9 kg.
- Average improvement in HbA1c of 18mmol/mol in type 2 diabetes.

Rather than giving patients advice, we gave information, and then asked patients if they were ready for change. The new diagnosis of diabetes is a strategic opportunity to offer dietary therapy as an alternative to lifelong medication. The point of initiating insulin is another such occasion. Given the choice and the information, not a single patient has chosen lifelong meds over dietary therapy in my GP practice. This has not only brought better patient health, but led to substantial savings, too. We now save over £50,000 each year on diabetes drugs compared to the U.K. average! Better health for less money.

In 2016, we collaborated with the clever folks at Diabetes.co.uk to produce a free on-line educational module. It offered fairly common-sense advice:

- Replace carbs with green vegetables and pulses [legumes].
- Enjoy olive oil, nuts, and other healthy saturated fats.
- Avoid added sugar.

In its first year 170,000 people have used it, in a backlash against official dietary advice by the National Health Service. After adopting this low-carbohydrate approach, patients lost an average of 8 kg. Over 70 percent of patients experienced improved blood glucose levels and an incredible 1 in 5 patients no longer required diabetic medication. Incredibly, these benefits were delivered entirely free in only ten weeks![33]

Dr. Osama Hamdy, the medical director of the Obesity Clinical Program at Harvard University's world famous Joslin Diabetes Center, has been prescribing low-carbohydrate diets extensively in the treatment of type 2 diabetes since 2005.[34] He writes, "It is clear that we made a major mistake in recommending the increase of carbohydrate loads." Increasing refined dietary carbohydrates naturally raises blood glucose in a situation where blood glucose is already toxically high. Dr. Elliott Joslin himself successfully treated so-called fatty diabetes (type 2 diabetes) with a diet that contained only 2 percent carbohydrates.

184

For more than a decade, guidelines from the Joslin Center's weight management program have advised clients to reduce their intake of refined carbohydrates to less than 40 percent of total calories. The result? Clients have lost more than 10,000 pounds of weight, improved their diabetes, and reduced their medications.

THREE RULES FOR REVERSING TYPE 2 DIABETES

ONCE WE UNDERSTAND how type 2 diabetes and insulin resistance develop, we can implement strategies that carry a reasonable chance of reversing it. Here are my top three food "rules" for reducing blood glucose, reducing insulin, and reversing type 2 diabetes.

Rule#1: Avoid fructose

The most important rule, without exception, is to eliminate all added sugars from your diet. Recall that insulin resistance is the result of fatty liver becoming overfilled and unable to accept more glucose. The most important determinant of fatty liver is not just carbohydrates, but the fructose contained in sucrose (table sugar) and high-fructose corn syrup.

Figure 14.6. The top dietary sources of fructose[35]

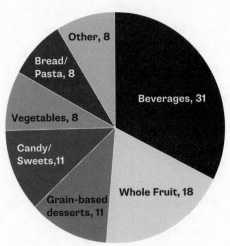

Remember that every single cell in the body can help disperse glucose, but the liver is the only organ that can metabolize fructose. Thus, fructose is many times more likely to cause fatty liver than glucose. Since sucrose is composed of equal amounts of glucose and fructose, it is the primary cause of fatty liver, bar none. Pure fructose is not commonly available, but may be found in some processed foods.

Some obvious foods to eliminate are sugar-sweetened beverages, including sodas, iced tea, sports drinks, mixed alcoholic drinks, juices, smoothies, coffee drinks, and "enhanced" water. These liquids are loaded with sugar. Cookies, cakes, desserts, muffins, cupcakes, and ice cream are other obvious sources.

Virtually all processed foods contain added sugars for the simple reason that they enhance flavor and texture at virtually no cost. Check the labels on meat products, where sugar is often added to the sauce or during processing. Sugar is often hidden in condiments (ketchup, relish), spaghetti/tomato sauces, flavored yogurts, salad dressings, barbecue sauces, applesauce, and spice mixes. Cereals and granola bars are usually very high in sugar too. And ask about your restaurant meals; sugar is often included in savory dishes because it's a cheap way to make all foods taste better.

What about fruit? The truth is there is no chemical difference between the fructose contained naturally in fruit and the fructose contained within sucrose. As with anything, *the dose makes the poison*. My best advice is to avoid eating excessive amounts of fruit, especially as many modern varieties are now available year-round and have been bred to be sweeter than in the past. Dried fruits are usually high in sugar, so you're probably best to avoid raisins, dried cranberries, fruit leathers, and the like.

What about artificial sweeteners? I advise patients to avoid all sweeteners, whether they contain calories or not. The logic is simple. If non-caloric sweeteners could truly reduce diabetes and obesity, then we would not have an epidemic on our hands. We have used these chemicals extensively in our food supply for decades and the empirical evidence is clear: artificial sweeteners are no better than sugar. Avoid them all.

Rule#2: Reduce refined carbohydrates and enjoy natural fats
Hyperinsulinemia and fatty liver are the key problems leading to the development of the metabolic syndrome, including obesity. Since refined carbohydrates, of all the food groups, cause the highest rise in insulin levels, it makes sense to eat less of them. Most processed products made with wheat, corn, rice, and potatoes belong in this group.

Reduce or avoid refined wheat products such as bread, pasta, waffles, muffins, cupcakes, and donuts. Limit processed corn products, such as popcorn, corn chips, and tortillas, and refined potato products, particularly french fries and potato chips. And eat white rice, which is also a refined carbohydrate, in small amounts. High-fructose corn syrup contains 55 percent fructose, which means it's sugar, not corn. It's found in many processed food products and should be avoided.

Remember that carbohydrates are not intrinsically bad foods. Many traditional societies ate diets heavy in carbohydrates and thrived. The refining process is the major problem. Removing the natural fats and protein and leaving behind a pure carbohydrate is not natural, and our bodies have not evolved to handle that change. Even many whole-wheat and whole-grain products are highly refined. The key is the insulin response to these foods, and whole, unrefined carbohydrates do not cause nearly the insulin response that white flour does.

Replace those refined carbohydrates with fatty fish, olive oil, avocados, and nuts. The natural saturated fats found in beef, pork, bacon, butter, cream, and coconuts are also healthy fats. Eggs are an excellent choice, as are most seafoods.

However, not all fats are benign. The industrially processed, highly refined seed oils that are high in omega-6 fat are *not* recommended because they can cause inflammation and adversely affect human health. These oils include sunflower, corn, canola, safflower, and vegetable oils. In particular, do not use these vegetable oils at high heat because they release harmful chemicals called aldehydes when heated. Stay away from deep-fried foods and all hydrogenated (trans) fats.

The diet I recommend has been called a low-carbohydrate, healthy-fat (LCHF) diet. It is designed to keep blood glucose low, decrease insulin, and therefore burn more fat. The result? Weight loss and an improvement in diabetes.

Rule#3: Eat real food

As I've said, there are good fats and bad fats. There are good carbohydrates and bad carbohydrates. What is the key distinguishing factor? Refining and processing.

Our bodies have had millennia to adapt to foods in their natural state. So some traditional societies, such as people living in the Far North, may eat an almost pure meat diet. And others, such as people living on the Japanese island of Okinawa, can eat a high-carbohydrate diet. Because these foods are not refined or processed, and because they contain little or no sugar, neither group has traditionally had trouble with high blood glucose, obesity, or type 2 diabetes. When traditional societies eating traditional diets begin to eat highly processed foods and sugar, however, obesity and type 2 diabetes follow closely behind.[36]

After all, you don't pick dinner rolls from the tree. You don't grow a bottle of vegetable oil. The most important rule of all is to just eat real food. If the food you are eating looks like it does when you see it in nature, it is probably good for you.

A FOURTH RULE, IN CASE THE FIRST THREE AREN'T ENOUGH

188 CERTAINLY, AVOIDING FRUCTOSE, eating a LCHF diet, and consuming real food is a great start, but these are often not enough to stop or reverse severe type 2 diabetes. The disease can take decades to develop, and so the vicious cycle of hyperinsulinemia and insulin resistance can

continue despite following all of the dietary rules. What if these simple dietary changes are not enough?

Like many solutions, the answer is not new. It's the oldest dietary intervention known to humans, its natural cleansing power has been harnessed by virtually all religions in the world, it's free, and it can be done anywhere. What am I talking about? The power of fasting.

INTERMITTENT FASTING

....

Again we keep this solemn fast
A gift of faith from ages past
ASCRIBED TO GREGORY THE GREAT, C. 540–604

FASTING, THE VOLUNTARY abstinence from food, has been known to cure diabetes for close to 100 years. Dr. Elliott Joslin, one of the most famous diabetes specialists in history, wrote about his experiences with fasting in 1916. He believed it was so obvious that fasting was helpful that studies would not even be necessary. For type 2 diabetes, it seems self-evident that if you don't eat, your blood glucose levels will drop and you will lose weight. As you lose weight, your type 2 diabetes will reverse. So, what's wrong with that?

As we've seen, the focus on dietary therapies for diabetes shifted with the momentous discovery of insulin. While insulin was indeed a miraculous cure for type 1, it was no panacea for type 2 diabetes. Interest in fasting disappeared as doctors focused on what would be their treatment mantra for the next century: drugs, drugs, and more drugs. When the American Diabetes Association says there is no cure for type 2 diabetes, what they mean is that there is no *drug* cure. However, these are two entirely different statements.

We've long known that bariatric surgery can reverse type 2 diabetes by inducing a sudden, severe caloric deficit, which drops insulin levels. Simply put, *bariatrics is surgically enforced fasting.* A study directly comparing the two approaches shows that fasting is actually better than surgery at lowering weight and reducing blood glucose.[1] Fasting produced almost *twice* the weight loss of bariatric surgery.

Food rationing across Europe during World Wars I and II restricted all foods, not specifically sugar. These austerity measures also acted like an enforced fast and reduced calories suddenly and severely. During that time, the mortality rate from diabetes dropped precipitously. Between the wars, as people went back to their accustomed eating habits, mortality returned to its usual high level. While food rationing is now a thing of the past in most countries, the point is simply this: strictly reducing food intake has the potential to entirely reverse type 2 diabetes. Once again, this seems self-evident. As you lose weight, type 2 diabetes disappears.

But surgery or wartime rationing is not the only way to create this sudden, severe caloric deprivation. We can simply stop eating. This is the time-tested, ancient healing tradition of fasting.

Remember that at its very core, type 2 diabetes is simply too much sugar in the body. Thus, reversal depends upon two things:

1. Stop putting sugar in.
2. Burn remaining sugar off.

A low-carbohydrate, healthy-fat diet reduces the incoming glucose load but does little to burn it off. Exercise may help, but the impact of compensation also limits its effectiveness. Further, exercise only benefits the skeletal muscles and not the fatty liver that is the cornerstone of this disease.

Intermittent fasting, though, can help simultaneously with both facets of diabetes reversal. Quite simply, it is the most powerful natural therapy available for type 2 diabetes. But can't you simply reduce your daily calorie intake to get the same effect? It sounds good, but the simple answer is no. *Continuous* mild calorie restriction is not at all the same as *intermittent*, severe restriction. Let me explain.

INTERMITTENT FASTING VERSUS CONTINUOUS
CALORIC REDUCTION
. . . .

DEATH VALLEY, CALIFORNIA, has an average temperature of 77 degrees Fahrenheit (25°C). Sounds perfect, doesn't it? Yet most residents would hardly call the temperature idyllic. Summer days are scorching hot and winter nights are uncomfortably cold.

Consider that jumping off a foot-high wall a thousand times is far different than jumping off a thousand-foot-high wall once. The difference between the two is literally the difference between life and death.

Would you prefer to experience seven gray, drizzling days with an inch of rain each, or six sunny, gorgeous days followed by a day of heavy thundershowers with 7 inches of rain?

The point, as Figure 15.1 shows, is that averages don't tell the whole story.

Figure 15.1. Averages don't tell the whole story

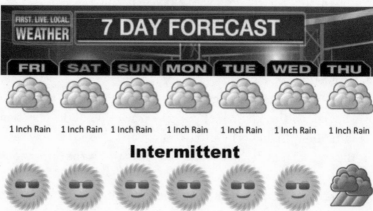

In all these examples, it's obvious that averages represent only one facet of the story. The frequency of the event is of paramount importance. So why would we assume that reducing 300 calories per day over seven days is the same as reducing 2100 calories over a single day? Constant caloric restriction is not the same as intermittent fasting. Each scenario provokes profoundly different hormonal responses in our body. The difference between the two is literally the difference between success and failure.

The portion-control strategy of constant caloric reduction is the most common dietary approach recommended to treat both weight loss and type 2 diabetes. For example, the American Diabetes Association's main dietary recommendation is "focus on diet, physical activity, and behavioral strategies to achieve a 500–750 kcal/day energy deficit."[2] It further advises patients to spread this reduction consistently throughout the day rather than all at once, and dieticians following this approach often counsel patients to eat four, five, or six times a day. In support of this reduction strategy, calorie labels are everywhere— on restaurant meals, packaged foods, and beverages. And if that's not enough, there are charts, apps, and hundreds of books to help us count calories. Even with all these aids, successful weight loss using this approach is as rare as humility in a grizzly bear.

After all, who *hasn't* tried the portion-control strategy? Does it work? Just about never. Data from the United Kingdom indicate that conventional advice succeeds in only 1 in 210 obese men and 1 in 124 obese women.[3] That is a failure rate of 99.5 percent, and that number is even worse for morbid obesity. So whatever else you may believe, portion control does *not* work. This is an empirically proven fact. Worse, it has also been proven in the bitter tears of a million believers.

But why doesn't it work? Because restricting calories causes a compensatory increase in hunger and a decrease in the body's metabolic rate. This effect derails weight-loss efforts and ultimately ends in failure. Intermittent fasting succeeds because it produces beneficial hormonal changes that chronic caloric deprivation does not. Most importantly, it reduces insulin and insulin resistance.

193

Remember the boy who cried wolf? Not crying wolf for a while will make the villagers listen. Crying wolf constantly but a little softer does not work. Resistance depends not only upon high insulin levels but also upon the persistence of those elevated levels. Intermittent fasting prevents the development of insulin resistance by creating extended periods of low insulin that maintain the body's sensitivity to insulin. This is the key to reversing prediabetes and type 2 diabetes.

Studies have directly compared daily caloric restriction with intermittent fasting, while keeping the weekly calorie intake similar.[4] Subjects ate a Mediterranean-style diet that included 30 percent fat, but some restricted a portion of their calories every day whereas others severely restricted their calories only two days a week and ate the full diet the rest of the time. That is, the groups differed only in how often they ate, but not in how many total weekly calories they consumed or the types of food they ate.

Over six months, the two groups showed no difference in the amount of weight and body fat loss between them, but an important difference between their insulin and insulin sensitivity levels. Remember, in the longer term insulin levels are the key driver of insulin resistance and obesity.

Those on a daily calorie-restricted diet saw their insulin levels drop but quickly reach a plateau. The intermittent fasting group, on the other hand, continued to reduce their fasting insulin levels, a key marker of improved insulin resistance, despite similar total caloric intake. Since type 2 diabetes is a disease of hyperinsulinemia and insulin resistance, the intermittent fasting strategy succeeded where caloric restriction did not. It was the *intermittency* of the diet that made it effective.

A recent thirty-two-week trial compared the portion-control strategy directly with intermittent fasting in obese adults.[6] The caloric reduction strategy was designed to subtract 400 calories per day from the estimated energy requirements of participants. The fasting group ate normally on eating days, but ate zero calories every other day.

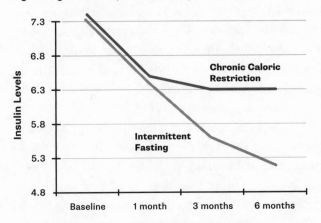

Figure 15.2. The impact of fasting on insulin resistance[5]

The most important conclusion was that fasting was a safe and effective therapy that anybody could reasonably follow. The fasting group not only lost more weight, but also almost twice as much of the more dangerous visceral fat. The portion-control group lost lean mass in addition to fat, but the fasting group did not. Lean mass percentage increased by 2.2 percent with fasting compared to only 0.5 percent with portion control. In other words, fasting is four times better at preserving lean mass. (So much for that old "fasting burns the muscle" myth.)

So why isn't fasting more popular, despite its proven success? One of the biggest deterrents is the starvation myth.

OVERCOMING THE STARVATION MYTH

The Biggest Loser is a long-running American TV reality show that pits obese contestants against one another in a bid to lose the most weight. The weight-loss regimen has two components: a calorie-restricted diet calculated to be approximately 70 percent of each contestant's energy requirements, typically 1200 to 1500 calories per day, combined with an intensive exercise regimen that is typically far in excess of two hours a day.[7]

195

This is the classic "Eat Less, Move More" approach endorsed by all the nutritional authorities, which is why *The Biggest Loser* diet scores well on the 2015 *U.S. News & World Report* ranking of best fast weight-loss diets.[8] And it does work—but only in the short term. When studied, average weight loss was 127 pounds over six months. That's amazing. Over the long-term, season two contestant Suzanne Mendonca said it best when she stated there is never a reunion show because "We're all fat again."[9]

These contestants' basal metabolic rates—the energy needed to keep the heart pumping, the lungs breathing, the brain thinking, the kidneys detoxing, and so on—dropped like a piano out of a twenty-story building. Over six months, their basal metabolism dropped by an average of 789 calories. Simply stated, they were burning 789 calories less each and every day. That's an almost insurmountable hurdle to continued weight loss.

As metabolism drops, weight loss plateaus. Chronic caloric reduction forces the body to shut down in order to match the lowered caloric intake. This compensation is sometimes called "starvation mode." Once expenditure drops below intake, the even more familiar weight regain begins. Goodbye reunion show. Even after six years, the metabolic rate does not recover.[10]

But this is not exactly news. This metabolic slowdown in response to caloric restriction has been scientifically proven for over fifty years. In the 1950s, Dr. Ancel Keys's famous Minnesota Starvation Experiment[11] placed volunteers on a diet of 1500 calories per day. Despite the study's name, this diet restricted calories by 30 percent over the subjects' usual diets—a degree of calorie restriction not dissimilar to many weight-loss diets recommended today. In response, the subjects' basal metabolic rate dropped about 30 percent. They felt cold, tired, and hungry. When they resumed their typical diet, all their weight came right back. Reversing type 2 diabetes relies upon burning off the body's excess glucose, so the daily calorie-restricted diet will not work.

The secret to long-term weight loss is to maintain your basal metabolism. So what *doesn't* put you into starvation mode? *Actual starvation!* Or at least the controlled version: intermittent fasting. Fasting triggers numerous hormonal adaptations that do *not* happen with simple caloric reduction. Insulin drops sharply, preventing insulin resistance. Noradrenaline rises, keeping metabolism high. Growth hormone rises, maintaining lean mass.

Controlled experiments prove this point. Over four days of continuous fasting, basal metabolism (measured as resting energy expenditure, REE) does not drop. Instead, it *increases* by 12 percent. The VO2, another measure of basal metabolism that tracks the amount of oxygen used per minute, similarly rises.[12] Many other studies have confirmed these findings. Twenty-two days of alternate daily fasting also did not result in any decrease in basal metabolic rate.[13]

Figure 15.3. Metabolic changes over four days of fasting[14]

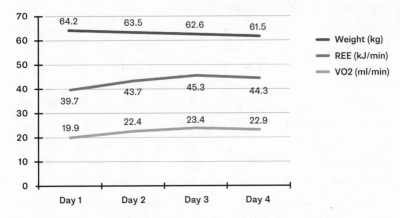

Remember the portion-control versus fasting study in the previous section? The portion-control strategy dropped basal metabolism by 76 calories per day. By contrast, fasting was not associated with any statistically significant drop in energy expenditure. In other words, daily caloric reduction causes starvation mode where fasting does not.

The study concluded: "Importantly, ADF (Alternate Daily Fasting) was not associated with an increased risk for weight regain." The importance of this statement will not be lost on anybody who has ever tried to lose weight. You can lose weight on virtually any diet, but *maintaining* this weight loss is the real battle.

Fasting works because it keeps basal metabolism high. Why? It's a survival mechanism. Imagine you are a cave dweller in the Stone Age. It's winter and food is scarce. If your body goes into starvation mode, you will not have the energy to go out and find food. Each day the situation will get worse and eventually you will die. The human species would have become extinct long ago if our bodies slowed down every time we didn't eat for a few hours.

During fasting, the body opens up its ample supply of stored food—body fat. Basal metabolism stays high, and instead of using food as our fuel, we use food our bodies have stored as body fat. After all, that's exactly why we stored it in the first place. Now we have enough energy to go out and hunt some woolly mammoth.

During fasting, we first burn glycogen stored in the liver. When that is finished, we use body fat. Oh hey, good news: there's plenty of fat stored here. Burn, baby, burn. And since there is plenty of fuel, there is no reason for basal metabolism to drop. That's the difference between long-term weight loss and a lifetime of despair. That's the knife edge between success and failure. Simply put, fasting provides beneficial hormonal changes that are entirely prevented by the constant intake of food, even when the calories in that food are reduced. It is the *intermittency* of the fasting that makes it so much more effective.

If we want our bodies to burn off the sugar that is causing type 2 diabetes, we need the fire of our basal metabolism to remain stoked. We can forge our new diabetes-free bodies in the crucible of fasting.

FASTING OR REDUCING CARBS: WHICH IS BETTER?

BOTH INTERMITTENT FASTING and low-carbohydrate, healthy-fat (LCHF) diets effectively reduce insulin, and thus can cause weight loss and reverse type 2 diabetes. Fasting lowers insulin maximally, so it is quite simply the quickest and most efficient method. Still, the very low–carbohydrate diet does remarkably well, giving you 71 percent of the benefits of the fasting without actual fasting.[15] Compared to the standard 55 percent carbohydrate diet, low-carbohydrate diets reduce insulin by roughly half, despite similar calorie intakes. Fasting reduces that by another 50 percent. That's power.

Notably, these studies demonstrate that the benefits of carbo-hydrate restriction on blood glucose were *not* simply due to calorie restriction. This is useful knowledge, considering how many health professionals keep parroting that "It's all about the calories." Actually, it's not. If it were true, then a plate of brownies would be as fatten-ing, and as likely to cause type 2 diabetes, as a kale salad with grilled salmon and olive oil, as long as the calories were equal. But this notion is clearly ridiculous.

The more we eat ultra-processed, insulin-stimulating food, the more we need to fast to bring those insulin levels back down. And *nothing* beats fasting for bringing down insulin. But should we fast or follow a LCHF diet? It's not a question of either/or. We can incorporate *both* fasting and a LCHF diet for maximal benefits.

If dietary interventions reduce both blood glucose and insulin for type 2 diabetes, why do we need medications at all? *We don't.* Type 2 diabetes is a dietary disease, and fixing the diet will reverse the disease.

FASTING FOR TYPE 2 DIABETES

FASTING ALLOWS US to naturally empty the sugar from our body (the sugar bowl). Once empty, any incoming sugar will no longer spill out into the blood, and we will no longer meet the criteria for diabetes. We will have reversed the disease.

As far back as 1916, Dr. Joslin reported the benefits of fasting for dia-betes. In the modern era, reports dating to 1969 confirm these benefits. Thirteen obese patients were hospitalized to treat their weight issues and were found incidentally to also have type 2 diabetes. They fasted for seventeen to ninety-nine days and averaged a 43-pound weight loss. Diabetes completely reversed, without exception. Interestingly, this reversal did not depend upon weight loss,[16] reflecting yet again that it is not total fat loss that matters, but ectopic fat loss.

Certain general principles apply to fasting with type 2 diabetes. How long it takes to reverse the disease depends on the intensity of the fasting regimen and the length of time you've had the disease. More intensive fasting will give quicker results, but if you have had type 2 diabetes for twenty years, it is unlikely to reverse in several months. It will take longer, though the exact time differs from patient to patient.

Fasting when taking medications

If you are taking medications, then you *must* speak with your physician before starting a fast. Diabetic medications are prescribed based on your current diet. If you change your diet without adjusting your medications, then you risk triggering hypoglycemic reactions, which are extremely dangerous. You may feel shaky, sweaty, or nauseated. In more severe cases, you could lose consciousness or even die. Carefully monitoring and adjusting your medications is essential.

Some diabetes drugs are more likely to cause hypoglycemia, especially insulin and sulfonylureas. Metformin, DPP-4 inhibitors, and SGLT2 inhibitors have a lower risk of hypoglycemia, so these are preferred. If you are taking medication for diabetes—and again, talk to your physician first—it's important to monitor your blood glucose frequently with a standard home monitor. Check your blood sugar at least twice a day and ideally up to four times a day on both fasting and non-fasting days. If you are not taking medication, this is not necessary. Blood glucose may drop slightly but should remain in the normal range.

Your physician can direct you on how to reduce or hold diabetic medications, and especially insulin, during fasting days. They can be taken on an as-needed basis when blood glucose goes too high. Modestly elevated blood glucose is not often a problem, since it can be expected to come down with fasting. In my Intensive Dietary

Management (IDM) program, for example, the target blood glucose is 8.0 to 10.0 mmol/L while fasting, if you are taking medication. This range is higher than the non-fasting norm. Mildly elevated blood glucose levels are not harmful in the short term, and this higher range creates a margin of safety to prevent the far more dangerous hypoglycemic reactions. I consider this to be an acceptable trade-off. The long-term goal is to successfully reduce and then stop all medications and still be able to maintain your sugars in the normal range.

If you are unsure whether to take medication or not, it is generally better to use less medication during fasting. If blood glucose rises too high, you can always take more medication to compensate. However, if you overmedicate and hypoglycemia develops, you must eat some sugar to treat it. That will break the fast and is counterproductive to reversing the diabetes. Again, consult with your doctor for guidance.

Medications unrelated to diabetes can often be taken as usual during fasting, though you must discuss them with your physician first. However, certain medications are best taken with food to avoid side effects. When taken on an empty stomach, metformin and iron supplements often cause diarrhea and stomach upset. Magnesium supplements can cause diarrhea. Aspirin may cause stomach pain and ulcers. Many aspirin preparations are coated to prevent this side effect but it may still occur.

Choosing a fasting regimen

No single fasting regimen is correct. The key is to choose the one that works best for you. Some people do well with an extended fast whereas others have better results with shorter, more frequent, fasts. You may need to try a few different fasting regimens to find the one that is most effective for you.

In my Intensive Dietary Management program, we often start with a thirty-six-hour fasting period three times per week for type 2 diabetes. During the eating periods, we prescribe a low-carbohydrate, high-fat diet. We provide strict medical supervision for patients, and frequent follow-up visits are essential. After they begin, we adjust the fasting schedule for each patient according to how they respond.

Some people will do a classic water-only fast, others a modified-fat fast, and still others a bone broth fast. It is important to drink fluids to stay hydrated and monitor yourself. If you feel ill at any point, you should stop and seek professional advice. Regardless of the regimen you choose, monitor your body weight, waist circumference, medications, and blood glucose. If everything is moving in the right direction, continue with the regimen. If your results stall or are getting worse, you must change the dietary regimen. Talk with your doctor about other options.

Everybody reacts differently to fasting. Some patients with long-standing diabetes completely reverse within several weeks. Others see very slow progress even with intensive fasting. Just because you are not getting the results you want does not necessarily mean you are doing it incorrectly or fasting isn't going to work for you. You may simply not have found the optimal regimen for you.

Intensifying the duration or frequency of your fasting regimen may improve the chances of getting results. Undertake shorter fasts more often. Extend a longer fast. Often it is useful to do a longer fast on a regular basis, say every three to six months. Or make your fast stricter, say, by shifting from a bone broth fast to a water-only fast.

If you find fasting difficult, it can be useful to closely monitor your diet and try to lower your dietary carbohydrates further.

What to expect when you start a fast: Dumping toxic load
Adjusting to a fast can take a bit of time. It's not unusual to get hunger pains or headaches or even to experience muscle cramps or skin irritations. These side effects are often signs that the body is dumping its toxic sugar load. Often, they will lessen and go away over a few weeks, but be sure to discuss them with your doctor. Another sign that the body is getting rid of its excess sugar is the dawn phenomenon.

What to expect after a period of fasting:
The dawn phenomenon

After a period of fasting, and especially in the morning, some people experience high blood glucose. This dawn phenomenon (DP), or dawn effect, was first described about thirty years ago. The DP is created by the circadian rhythm. Just before awakening (around 4 am), the body secretes higher levels of adrenaline, growth hormone, glucagon, and cortisol to prepare for the upcoming day. Adrenaline gives our body some energy. Growth hormone helps repair and synthesize new protein. Glucagon helps move glucose from storage into the blood so it's ready to use as energy. Cortisol, the stress hormone, gets us ready for activity. After all, we are never quite so relaxed as in deep sleep. This normal circadian hormonal surge tells the liver to start pushing out some glucose and generally activates the body. It's a good ol' fashioned hormonal kick in the ass, so to speak.

These hormones are secreted in a pulsatile manner, peaking in the early morning hours then falling to low levels during the day. In nondiabetic situations where there is no need to manage blood glucose artificially, the DP is a normal occurrence, but most people miss it because the magnitude of the rise is very small.

In about 75 percent of type 2 diabetics, however, it shows up as a noticeable spike in blood glucose levels early in the morning. The severity varies widely and occurs whether patients are being treated with insulin or not because the huge fatty liver wants desperately to deflate itself. As soon as it gets the signal, sugar comes whooshing out of the liver and into the blood. Like the overinflated balloon, the liver puts forth prodigious amounts of sugar in order to relieve itself of this toxic sugar burden. As an analogy, think about a time when you really, really needed to urinate. You had drunk too much water and there was no bathroom nearby. When the time finally came to pee, there was no stopping that large, fast flow. That's the dawn phenomenon.

The same phenomenon exists during extended fasts, which induce the same hormonal changes as shorter overnight fasts. Insulin drops,

203

so the liver releases some of its stored sugar and fat. This is natural. In type 2 diabetes, all that sugar pent up inside the fatty liver whooshes out too quickly and shows up, like an uninvited guest, as glucose in the blood. Even if you have not eaten for a while, the body will still release its stored sugar.

Is this a bad thing? No, not at all. We are merely moving the sugar from storage in the liver, where we could not see it, into the blood where it becomes visible. The dawn phenomenon, or higher blood glucose during fasting, does not mean you are doing anything wrong. It's a normal occurrence. It just means that you have more work to do to burn off all the stored sugar in the body.

If your blood glucose rises during fasting, ask yourself where that glucose came from. The only possibility is that it came from your own body. You are simply moving some stored food energy out from the body and into the blood for you to use.

TOWARD A CURE: PREVENTION, TREATMENT, ERADICATION

IMAGINE A WORLD without obesity, type 2 diabetes, and metabolic syndrome. No more diabetic kidney disease. No more diabetic eye disease. No more diabetic nerve damage. No more diabetic foot ulcers. No more diabetic infections. Fewer heart attacks. Fewer strokes. Fewer cancers. No more need for diabetic medications. Can we really dare to dream? *Yes, we can.*

With a new, deeper understanding of type 2 diabetes and its effective treatments, we can eradicate this disease. We can reverse type 2 diabetes, completely naturally, completely without cost, completely without surgery—*completely.* Equally important, we can also now forestall it.

204 The northern city of Da Qing in China's Heilongjiang Province gained national prominence as the site of China's most productive oil field and one of its richest cities. But, as emphasis shifts to cleaner energy, Da Qing is becoming known globally for a completely separate reason: its *prevention* of type 2 diabetes.

In 1986, the World Health Organization funded the China Da Qing Diabetes Prevention Outcomes Study,[17] a randomized, controlled trial of 577 Chinese adults with prediabetes. The main dietary intervention was to increase intake of vegetables and reduce consumption of alcohol and sugar. Counselors also encouraged lifestyle measures, including more physical activity.

Active intervention over six years reduced the incidence of diabetes by a stunning 43 percent, and this benefit was sustained over twenty years. The onset of type 2 diabetes was delayed by an average of 3.6 years. The cardiovascular death rate fell from 20 percent to only 1 percent. Professor Nicholas Wareham of University of Cambridge commented that the study was a "real breakthrough, showing that lifestyle intervention can reduce the risk of long-term cardiovascular consequences of diabetes."[18]

Multiple studies of lifestyle interventions similar to ones in Da Qing have shown exactly the same benefit. Although the dietary intervention varies depending upon the study, most focus upon weight loss. In the United States, the Diabetes Prevention Program reduced the incidence of type 2 diabetes by 58 percent[19] and sustained the benefits for ten years.[20] The Indian Diabetes Prevention Programme reduced the incidence of type 2 diabetes by almost 30 percent.[21] The Finnish Diabetes Prevention Study reported a 58 percent reduction.[22] A Japanese trial reduced progression by 67 percent.[23]

All these successful trials shared one common factor of overriding importance. They all used lifestyle interventions, *not medications*. So type 2 diabetes is not only a treatable disease, but a preventable one.

REVERSING AND PREVENTING TYPE 2 DIABETES NATURALLY: A BRAVE NEW WORLD

OBESITY, FATTY LIVER, metabolic syndrome, and type 2 diabetes are the twenty-first-century equivalents of the Bubonic plague that killed an estimated fifty million people in Asia, Europe, and Africa during the fourteenth century. Despite advances in computer technology, genetic engineering, and molecular biology, the problem only grows worse and has now engulfed the entire world, reaching across all genetic boundaries. It's time to stop pretending type 2 diabetes is a chronic and progressive disease, and it's time to stop treating it that way. Clearly type 2 diabetes is a dietary and lifestyle disease. To pretend otherwise is pure self-deception.

But here's what is important. *A dietary disease requires a dietary treatment.* And since weight gain clearly plays a prominent role in the development of type 2 diabetes, weight loss must similarly play a large role in its reversal. We know that bariatric surgery, very low-carbohydrate diets, and fasting are well-known treatments for type 2 diabetes and they are proven to cure. We also know that insulin, oral hypoglycemics, and low-fat diets can lower blood glucose but do nothing to cure type 2 diabetes.

Figure 15.4. Dietary disease; dietary treatment

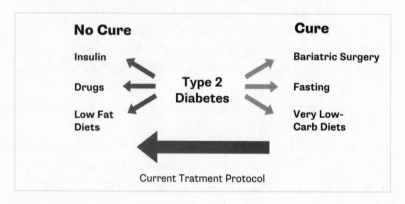

The treatments that cure all show one common characteristic. They lower insulin. Since type 2 diabetes is a disease of hyperinsulinemia, it is only logical that these treatments are beneficial. And what do all the treatments that do *not* cure type 2 diabetes have in common? They raise insulin. And in fact, using these treatments *worsens* diabetes over time.

Again, let's juxtapose two incontrovertible facts:

Fact #1: Type 2 diabetes is a reversible disease.

Fact #2: Virtually all conventionally treated patients get worse.

Unfortunately, there is only one conclusion. The conventional treatment recommended by virtually every doctor in the world is not correct. This is terrific news! Why? Because it means we can change its natural history. It means the doorway to a diabetes-free world has just opened.

We can prevent and cure not just type 2 diabetes but the entire metabolic syndrome completely and utterly with knowledge alone. Not the latest and greatest invention, but the tried and true. The oldest lifestyle interventions known to humans: a LCHF diet and intermittent fasting. A world freed from the chains of type 2 diabetes awaits. Like dreams waiting to be dreamt, a cure beckons. We need only to take those first few, brave steps to cross the threshold. The journey toward better health, free of obesity and type 2 diabetes, now begins.

ALBERTO

Alberto, 70, had a seventeen-year history of type 2 diabetes and had been taking insulin in ever-increasing doses for nearly ten of them. His A1C was 7.7% and he was on 160 units of insulin a day, as well as sitagliptin. Alberto also had a history of chronic kidney disease, hypertension, and sleep apnea.

When he entered the IDM program, Alberto started on a low-carbohydrate, healthy-fat diet with 24 to 42 hours of fasting, five days per week. Within a month, he completely stopped all his medications, including insulin; his blood glucose was better than ever, with his A1C at 7.3%. Just three months into the program, Alberto has lost 24 pounds and is well on his way to regaining his health.

LANA

Lana was just 18 years old when she was diagnosed with type 2 diabetes. For thirteen years, she took blood-glucose-lowering medications. She began taking insulin as well when she became pregnant at age 31. Even after her pregnancy, her A1C was 7.2% and her doctor continued her on 82 units of insulin a day in addition to metformin.

When Lana entered the IDM program, she started with a seven-day fast. By the end of that week, her sugars had normalized and she was able to stop taking all her medications; she has not resumed them since. She then settled into a routine of fasting for 42 hours, two to three times per week. After a year on the program, Lana has lost 55 pounds, including 33 cm around her waist, and her A1C has dropped to 6.1%.

AFTERWORD

········

DESPITE THE TITLE of this book and its in-depth exploration of type 2 diabetes, it may surprise you to learn that I do not truly consider this book to be about diabetes. "What?" I can hear you protesting. "Almost every word in this book discusses diabetes!" No, my friend, this book is truly about *hope*.

I hope we can eradicate type 2 diabetes within a generation. I hope we can erase all the diseases associated with metabolic syndrome. I hope we can recover all the associated costs, both in dollars and human suffering. I hope we can accomplish these goals without drugs and without surgery, using only knowledge as our weapon.

HOW IT BEGAN: MY JOURNEY TO HOPE

IN A SENSE, this book parallels my own journey. I entered medical school at the University of Toronto just after I turned nineteen. Once I finished medical school, I trained conventionally in internal medicine and then I spent two years completing my specialty training in kidney disease (nephrology) at Cedars-Sinai Medical Center in Los Angeles. Since 2001, I have practiced clinical nephrology in Toronto, which means that I have now spent more than half of my life in the study of medicine. During my entire education, I received virtually no training in nutrition and certainly did not see it as my area of specialization.

As a kidney specialist, I know that type 2 diabetes is, by far, the biggest cause of kidney disease. I have seen many patients with mild forms of the disease and treated them exactly as I, as well as countless other doctors, had been taught. I prescribed medications to keep their blood glucose low. When that didn't work, I prescribed insulin. When that didn't work, I kept right on increasing the dose. Every medical school and medical association taught, and still teaches, that tight blood glucose control was the key to managing type 2 diabetes.

After treating thousands of patients over decades, it gradually dawned on me that none of these diabetes medications actually made any real difference to the health of patients. Sure, the medical schools *said* these drugs improved patient health, but any benefits were imperceptible. Whether these patients took their medications or not, they still progressed to more and more severe forms of disease. Their kidneys failed. They had heart attacks. They got strokes. They went blind. They needed amputations.

Once their kidneys failed, I would start them on dialysis. I have seen more diabetic foot infections, diabetic ulcers, heart attacks, and strokes than I can count. Even if they made a statistical difference, the medicines I prescribed made no real clinical difference. I suspected that we only *thought* these medicines made a difference because we were being *told* they made a difference.

Clinical trial evidence finally caught up with real-world experience in 2008. That year, the results of the landmark randomized ACCORD and ADVANCE studies were released, followed shortly by the ORIGIN and VADT studies. Confirming perfectly my experience treating patients, the studies proved conclusively that using blood glucose-lowering medications for type 2 diabetes was useless.

Doctors like me were certainly prescribing a lot of medications, but these drugs provided no protection against heart disease, stroke, death, eye disease, or kidney disease. If anything, insulin seemed to make things worse, not better. Now it was a proven fact. This core principle of treating type 2 diabetes—taught in every medical school in the world—had just been disproven.

The entire treatment paradigm of type 2 diabetes needed to change. We had to incorporate this new hard-won knowledge to gain a newer, more complete understanding. However, what happened next was unfortunate, even if it was entirely predictable. Rather than developing new paradigms of insulin resistance, which could lead to more effective treatments, we clung to the old, failed paradigms because it is far easier to ignore an inconvenient truth than to face it. So we kept on giving the exact same medications, using the same treatments and getting the same poor outcomes. Same old thinking, same old results. Insanity, as Albert Einstein would have said. Patients continued to get sick and die.

Breaking paradigms is hard work. We were so intent on treating the high blood glucose that we forgot to treat the diabetes. If losing weight was the key to reversing diabetes, how could medications like insulin, which causes weight gain, be beneficial? We made no serious attempts to look for explanations. The reality was troublesome, so it was easier for doctors and researchers to live in a pretend world where these medications were the correct treatment for diabetes.

NEW PARADIGMS FOR OBESITY

WHILE DIABETES RESEARCHERS may not have been looking for alternatives, new paradigms were forming in the field of obesity medicine. Interesting studies were being published about the effectiveness and dangers of low-carbohydrate diets. In the late 1990s, the low-carbohydrate Atkins-styled diets enjoyed a huge surge of popularity. Health professionals like me and most other physicians were aghast, positive that these high-fat Atkins-styled diets would cause heart disease. A number of trials were launched in the early 2000s to prove this precise point.

Then a funny thing happened, or rather didn't happen: anything bad. Those predictions that the high-fat diet would cause high cholesterol levels and clog arteries were wrong. Actually, the opposite was true. Not only did patients lose weight, their entire metabolic profile improved, including their cholesterol levels. Trial after trial showed that these low-carbohydrate, high-fat diets were safe and effective. A few years later, in 2006, the Women's Health Initiative, the largest randomized dietary trial ever done, proved beyond a doubt that low-fat diets did not protect against heart disease, strokes, or cancer. Worse, the calorie restriction also did not cause weight loss or reduce type 2 diabetes. The entire foundation of modern nutritional advice was completely shattered.

The entire treatment paradigm of obesity needed to change. Yet once again, physicians around the world continued to practice as if nothing had changed. We clung to old, failed paradigms like a life raft. We continued to preach a low-fat diet. We continued to advise people to "Eat Less and Move More." We got the same poor results, and patients continued to become obese and get sick. Same old thinking, same old results. Yes, insanity.

Not satisfied with these two deep paradoxes, I started to look for answers starting from ground zero. I made no assumptions about what caused obesity or type 2 diabetes. This was the most important step. Breaking free of all the old assumptions allowed me to see, all of a sudden, how certain facts, hidden in plain view, became obvious.

MY SEARCH FOR ANSWERS: ALWAYS START WITH "WHY"

THE QUESTION OF causality has always intrigued me. I like to understand the mechanism of disease, the question of "why." Obesity is no different. "Why do people get fat?" I wondered. This question is absolutely critical because without understanding how people get fat I could not understand how to effectively treat the disease.

I had never really considered this important question, and it turns out that virtually nobody else had either. We all thought we already knew the answer. Too many calories cause obesity. If that were true, then reducing calories should cause weight loss. *Except it doesn't.* The failure rate of caloric reduction diets was astronomically high. My search for the true underlying cause led ultimately to my recognition that a hormonal imbalance, predominantly of insulin, is the key to obesity. I detail this process in my first book, *The Obesity Code.*

But this answer only led me to another paradox. If too much insulin was causing obesity, then why would I, as a physician, prescribe insulin to overweight type 2 diabetics? It would only make things worse. Insulin was the *problem*, not the answer.

Interestingly, my patients already knew. "Doc," they would say, "you've always told me to lose weight but now you give me insulin, which has made me put on 50 pounds. How is that good?" The answer was that it was not good; it was absurd.

My next question, then, was "Why does type 2 diabetes develop?" Again, always start with "why?" Everybody agreed that elevated insulin resistance caused the high blood glucose that was the hallmark of type 2 diabetes. But what caused the elevated insulin resistance? This was the true question that I desperately needed to answer.

The key insight came from understanding obesity. Too much insulin causes obesity, so it is logical that too much insulin could also cause insulin resistance and type 2 diabetes. That obesity and type 2 diabetes were manifestations of the same disease, and simply flip sides to the same coin, explained perfectly how these two diseases were so closely related.

Albert Einstein once said, "When you have eliminated the impossible, whatever remains, however improbable, must be the truth." If the problem was too much insulin, then the answer was simplicity itself. Lower insulin. But how? No drugs at the time effectively did that. The solution was to go back to the basics. As a dietary disease, it required a dietary solution, not a pharmaceutical one. Since refined carbohydrates stimulate insulin the most and dietary fat the least, the obvious solution was to eat a low-carbohydrate, high-fat diet.

INTENSIVE DIETARY MANAGEMENT: SPREAD THE WORD

IN 2011, I established the Intensive Dietary Management program in Scarborough, Ontario, along with Megan Ramos, a medical researcher long interested in this exact problem. Together, we counseled patients, many with type 2 diabetes, on how to follow a low-carbohydrate, high-fat diet. I believed and hoped they would improve their health.

The results were a disaster. Nobody lost weight. Nobody got better. A review of my patients' diet diaries revealed they were eating lots of bread, noodles, and rice. They had misunderstood these foods as being part of a low-carbohydrate diet. Having followed a low-fat diet for most of their lives, this new regimen was entirely foreign to them, and they didn't know what to eat. I needed to find a simpler solution.

One day, a friend told me about her "cleanses," and immediately I rolled my eyes. Like most people, my gut reaction was that fasting would never work. But what, really, was wrong with fasting? I was intrigued enough to start investigating the medical literature, most of which was decades old. The more I understood the physiology, the more I realized there was simply no reason that fasting couldn't be used successfully as a therapeutic intervention. After all, it was the oldest and perhaps the simplest solution. I started to guide patients through diet and fasting regimes. This time, the results were completely different.

Some of the success stories were almost unbelievable. Patients who had been taking high doses of insulin for decades would eliminate all their medications in a matter of weeks. My patients lost significant weight and kept it off. Interestingly, many patients reported that it was much, much easier to follow the program than they had anticipated. They expected their hunger would grow unimaginably intense, but the opposite was true. As they continued fasting, their hungers and cravings often dissipated like a morning fog. Some thought their stomach had shrunk. They expected fasting would leave them weak and unable to concentrate, but the opposite was true. Women who had barely had enough energy to walk in the door would come running in. Their husbands said they couldn't keep up with them any longer.

216

As the pieces came together, I began lecturing to both patients and physicians around Toronto. I posted my six-part lecture "The Aetiology of Obesity" series on YouTube[1] and started my blog, "Intensive Dietary Management"[2] to share my findings with the general public. One night, I gave a lecture to a group of specialist physicians about obesity. After the first hour-long lecture, they were so interested in the new paradigms that I gave a second lecture. One of those physicians later contacted Rob Sanders of Greystone Books, who asked me to write a book about obesity and type 2 diabetes. Rob has been hugely supportive from the beginning, for which I am very grateful.

There was too much material for a single book. To properly address the misconceptions of obesity and type 2 diabetes and lay the foundation for treatment, the book would have been 800 pages—intimidating just to look at. The natural solution was to divide this material into two books. *The Obesity Code*, published in 2016, set the stage for the deeper understanding of type 2 diabetes in this book. Together, they enable readers to naturally reverse obesity and type 2 diabetes.

Every single day, I see patients whose type 2 diabetes is reversing, patients who are losing weight and getting healthier. This is the reason I became a doctor! I want to help people regain their health, and I want to give people hope that they can indeed defeat obesity and type 2 diabetes, completely naturally. That's perfect, because patients also do not want to be sick or take medications. It's a win-win situation.

HOPE FOR THE FUTURE

TYPE 2 DIABETES is currently the leading cause of blindness, kidney failure, amputations, heart attacks, strokes, and cancer. But it doesn't have to be our future. The pages of *The Obesity Code* and *The Diabetes Code* contain the knowledge to reverse type 2 diabetes. This is not the end, but only the beginning. A new hope arises. A new dawn breaks.

APPENDIX:
TWO SAMPLE WEEK-LONG
MEAL PLANS

....

EACH OF THESE meal plans, designed by my colleague Megan Ramos at Intensive Dietary Management (www.IDMprogram. com), consists of three 30- to 36-hour fasts done on three alternate days of the week. During the fasting period, you do not take any meals. You can consume fasting fluids such as water, green tea, herbal tea, and coffee during this time.

In Sample 1, if you begin your 36-hour fast after dinner (7:30 p.m.) on Sunday night, you would not eat again until breakfast on Tuesday morning (7:30 a.m.). In other words, you will not consume breakfast, lunch, dinner, or any snacks during your fasting days. On non-fasting days, you can eat meals and snacks as usual.

In Sample 2, if you begin your 30-hour fast after lunch (12:30 p.m.) on Sunday, you would not eat again until dinner (6:30 p.m.) on Monday night. Again, you will not consume any food during your fasting period but you are encouraged to stay hydrated by drinking plenty of fasting fluids. This schedule incorporates slightly shorter fasting periods, with the advantage of eating at least one meal per day. If you are taking medications that must be taken with food, this schedule may be useful.

The following meal plans provide two sample schedules for a

30- to 36-hour fasting regimen complemented by a low-carbohydrate, healthy-fat diet. Remember to consult with your doctor before you begin this or any new regimen. Sparkling or still water, green teas, or herbal teas are excellent drinks to accompany these meals.

SAMPLE 1:

MEAL PLAN FOR A 36-HOUR FASTING PERIOD

MEAL	Sunday	Monday	Tuesda
Breakfast	Mini Bacon-Wrapped Egg Frittatas	FAST	Western Omele with Sausage
Lunch	Arugula and Prosciutto Salad	FAST	Chicken Drum sticks Wrapped Bacon with Slic of Celery and Carrots
Dinner	Almond Flour and Pork Rind–Breaded Chicken Tenders	FAST	Beef Stir Fry

ednesday	Thursday	Friday	Saturday
ST	Bacon, Scrambled Eggs, and Avocado	FAST	Coconut Flour Pancakes with Whipped Cream and Berries
ST	Chicken-Stuffed Bell Peppers	FAST	Pear and Arugula Salad with Pine Nuts
ST	BBQ Shrimp Skewers	FAST	Pulled Pork Sliders on Almond Flour Buns

SAMPLE 2:
MEAL PLAN FOR A 30-HOUR FASTING PERIOD

MEAL	Sunday	Monday	Tuesday
Breakfast	Scrambled Eggs, Smoked Salmon, and Avocado	FAST	Hard-Boiled Eggs, Cauliflowe Hash Browns, ar Asparagus
Lunch	Lemon Butter and Pepper Chicken Wings, Celery, and Carrots	FAST	Chicken "Breade in Pork Rinds wi Green Beans
Dinner	FAST	Grilled Salmon with Garden Salad	FAST

ednesday	Thursday	Friday	Saturday
ST	Mushroom Omelet	FAST	Chia Pudding
ST	Steak Fajitas	FAST	Tomato, Cucumber, and Avocado Salad
chini Pasta vocado Pesto h Stir-fried etables	FAST	Ginger Chicken Lettuce Cups with Baby Bok Choy	FAST

ENDNOTES

....

Foreword

1. For the rest of the foreword, diabetes will refer exclusively to type 2 diabetes.

2. Phinney S, Volek J. The art and science of low carbohydrate living: an expert guide to making the life-saving benefits of carbohydrate restriction sustainable and enjoyable. Miami: Beyond Obesity LLC, 2011; Bernstein R, Diabetes type II: Living a long, healthy life through blood sugar normalization, 1st ed. New Jersey: Prentice Hall Trade, 1990, plus subsequent publications.

3. Remote care promotes low carbohydrate diet adherence and glycemic control allowing medication reduction in type 2 diabetes—abstract. Virta Health blog. 2017 Jun 14. Available from: http://blog.virtahealth.com/remote-care-promotes-low-carbohydrate-diet-adherence-and-glycemic-control-allowing-medication-reduction-in-type-2-diabetes-abstract/. Accessed 2017 Jun 20. Six months results are published here: McKenzie L et al. A novel intervention including individualized nutritional recommendations reduces hemoglobin A1C level, medication use, and weight in type 2 diabetes. JMIR Diabetes. 2017; 2(1): e5. doi:10.2196/diabetes.6981.

4. Hallberg S, Hamdy O. Before you spend $26,000 on weight-loss surgery, do this. New York Times. 2016 Sep 10. Available from: https://www.nytimes.com/2016/09/11/opinion/sunday/before-you-spend-26000-on-weight-loss-surgery-do-this.html?_r=0. Accessed on 2017 Jun 20; Advice on diabetes. New York Times. 2016 Sep 20. Available from: https://www.nytimes.com/2016/09/21/opinion/advice-on-diabetes.html. Accessed on 2017 Jun 20.

Chapter 1

1. Sanders LJ. From Thebes to Toronto and the 21st century: an incredible journey. Diabetes Spectrum. 2002 Jan; 15(1): 56–60.

2. Lakhtakia R. The history of diabetes mellitus. Sultan Qaboos Univ Med J. 2013 Aug; 13(3): 368–370.

3. Karamanou M, et al. Apollinaire Bouchardat (1806–1886): founder of modern Diabetology. Hormones. 2014 Apr–Jun; 13(2): 296–300.

4. Mazur A. Why were "starvation diets" promoted for diabetes in the pre-insulin period? Nutr J. 2011; 10(1): 23. doi: 10.1186/1475-2891-10-23. Accessed 2017 Jun 6.

5. Franz, MJ. The history of diabetes nutrition therapy. Diabetes Voice. 2004 Dec; 49: 30–33.

6. Joslin EP. The treatment of diabetes mellitus. Can Med Assoc J. 1916 Aug; 6(8): 673–684.

7. Bliss M. The Discovery of Insulin. 2015 Aug 19. Historica Canada. Available from: http://www.thecanadianencyclopedia.ca/en/article/the-discovery-of-insulin/. Accessed 2017 Jun 6.

8. Furdell EL. Fatal thirst: diabetes in Britain until insulin. Boston: Brill; 2009. p. 147.

9. Himsworth HP. Diabetes mellitus: its differentiation into insulin-sensitive and insulin-insensitive types. Lancet. 1936; 1: 127–130.

10. Joslin EP. The unknown diabetic. Postgraduate Medicine. 1948; 4(4): 302–306.

11. US Dept of Health and Human Services and US Dept of Agriculture. Executive summary. 2015–2020 Dietary guidelines for Americans. Available from: http://health.gov/dietaryguidelines/2015/guidelines/executive-summary/. Accessed 2017 Jun 6.

12. Siri-Tarino PW, et al. Meta-analysis of prospective cohort studies evaluating the association of saturated fat with cardiovascular disease. Am J Clin Nutr. 2010; 91(3): 535–546, doi: 10.3945/ajcn.2009.27725. Accessed 2017 Jun 6.; Mente A, et al. A systematic review of the evidence supporting a causal link between dietary factors and coronary heart disease. Arch Intern Med. 2009; 169(7): 659–669.

13. Centers for Disease Control and Prevention. Prevalence of overweight, obesity, and extreme obesity among adults: United States, trends 1960–1962 through 2007–2008. 2011 Jun 6. Available from: http://www.cdc.gov/nchs/data/hestat/obesity_adult_07_08/obesity_adult_07_08.htm. Accessed 2015 Apr 26. Used with permission.

14. World Health Organization. Global report on diabetes. 2016. Available from: http://apps.who.int/iris/bitstream/10665/204871/1/9789241565257_eng.pdf. Accessed 2017 Jun 6.

15. Pinhas-Hamiel O, Zeitler P. The global spread of type 2 diabetes mellitus in children and adolescents. J Pediatr. 2005; 146(5): 693–700. doi: 10.1016/j.jpeds.2004.12.042. Accessed 2017 Jun 6.

16. Centers for Disease Control and Prevention. Number (in Millions) of Civilian, Non-Institutionalized Persons with Diagnosed Diabetes, United States, 1980-2014. Available from: https://www.cdc.gov/diabetes/statistics/prev/national/figpersons. htm. Accessed 2017 Jun 6. Used with permission.

17. Tabish SA. Is diabetes becoming the biggest epidemic of the twenty-first century? Int J Health Sci. 2007; 1(2): 5–8.

18. Xu Y, et al. Prevalence and control of diabetes in Chinese adults. JAMA. 2013; 310(9): 948–958.

19. International Diabetes Federation. IDF diabetes atlas, 7th edition. 2015. p. 14. Available from: www.idf.org/diabetesatlas. Accessed 2017 Jan 15.

20. Menke A, et al. Prevalence of and trends in diabetes among adults in the United States, 1988–2012. JAMA. 2015; 314(10): 1021–1029.

21. Polonsky KS. The past 200 years in diabetes. N Engl J Med 2012; 367(14): 1332–1340.

Chapter 2

1. American Diabetes Association. Standards of medical care in diabetes—2016. Diabetes Care. 2016; 39(Suppl. 1): S13–S22.

2. Zhang X, et al. A1C level and future risk of diabetes: a systematic review. Diabetes Care. 2010; 33(7): 1665–1673.

3. Van Bell TL, et al. Type 1 diabetes: etiology, immunology, and therapeutic strategies. Phys Rev 2011; 91(1): 79–118.

4. Joslin's diabetes mellitus, 14th edition. Boston: Lippincott Williams & Wilkins; 2005. p. 399.

5. Type 1 diabetes. New York Times. 2014 July 21. Available from: http://www.nytimes.com/health/guides/disease/type-1-diabetes/complications.html. Accessed 2017 Jun 6.

6. Rosenbloom AL, et al. Type 2 diabetes in children and adolescents. Pediatr Diabetes 2009; 10(Suppl. 12): 17–32.

7. Haines L, et al. Rising incidence of type 2 diabetes in children in the U.K. Diabetes Care. 2007; 30(5): 1097–1101.

8. Grinstein G, et al. Presentation and 5-year follow-up of type 2 diabetes mellitus in African-American and Caribbean-Hispanic adolescents. Horm Res 2003; 60(3): 121–126.

9. Pinhas-Hamiel O, Zeitler P. The global spread of type 2 diabetes mellitus in

children and adolescents. J Pediatr. 2005; 146(5): 693–700. doi: 10.1016/j.jpeds. 2004.12.042. Accessed 2017 Jun 6.

Chapter 3

1. U.S. Department of Health and Human Services. National Diabetes Fact Sheet, 2011. Available from: http://www.cdc.gov/diabetes/pubs/pdf/ndfs_2011.pdf. Accessed 2017 Jun 6.

2. Fong DS, et al. Diabetic retinopathy. Diabetes Care. 2004; 27(10): 2540–2553.

3. Keenan HA, et al. Clinical factors associated with resistance to microvascular complications in diabetic patients of extreme disease duration: the 50-year medalist study. Diabetes Care. 2007; 30(8):1995–1997.

4. National Institute of Diabetes and Digestive and Kidney Diseases. Diabetic kidney disease. 2016 Jul. Available from: http://www.niddk.nih.gov/health-information/health-topics/kidney-disease/kidney-disease-of-diabetes/Pages/facts.aspx. Accessed 2017 Jun 6.

5. National Institute of Diabetes and Digestive and Kidney Diseases. Adjusted prevalence rates of ESRD. Available from: http://www.niddk.nih.gov/health-information/health-statistics/Pages/kidney-disease-statistics-united-states.aspx. Accessed 2017 Jun 6. Used with permission.

6. Adler AI, et al. Development and progression of nephropathy in type 2 diabetes: The United Kingdom Prospective Diabetes Study (UKPDS 64). Kidney Int. 2003; 63(1): 225–232.

7. National Institute of Diabetes and Digestive and Kidney Diseases. Nerve damage (diabetic neuropathies). 2013 Nov. Available from: http://www.niddk.nih.gov/health-information/health-topics/Diabetes/diabetic-neuropathies-nerve-damage-diabetes/Pages/diabetic-neuropathies-nerve-damage.aspx. Accessed 2017 Jun 6.

8. Fowler MJ. Microvascular and macrovascular complications of diabetes. Clin Diabetes. 2008; 26(2): 77–82.

9. Boulton AJ, et al. Diabetic neuropathies: a statement by the American Diabetes Association. Diabetes Care. 2005; 28(4): 956–962.

10. Maser RE, et al. The association between cardiovascular autonomic neuropathy and mortality in individuals with diabetes: a meta-analysis. Diabetes Care. 2003; 26(6): 1895–1901.

11. Kannel WB, et al. Diabetes and cardiovascular disease: the Framingham study. JAMA. 1979; 241(19): 2035–2038.

12. American Heart Association. Cardiovascular disease & diabetes. 2015 Aug. Available from: http://www.heart.org/HEARTORG/Conditions/More/Diabetes/WhyDiabetesMatters/Cardiovascular-Disease-Diabetes_UCM_313865_Article.jsp/#.WZYRWK3MXE4. Accessed 2017 Jun 6.

13. Gu K, et al. Diabetes and decline in heart disease mortality in U.S. adults. JAMA. 1999; 281(14): 1291–1297.

14. Beckman JA, et al. Diabetes and atherosclerosis: epidemiology, pathophysiology and management. JAMA. 2002; 287(19): 2570–2581.

15. Air EL, Kissela BM. Diabetes, the metabolic syndrome, and ischemic stroke: epidemiology and possible mechanisms. Diabetes Care. 2007; 30(12): 3131–3140.

16. Banerjee C, et al. Duration of diabetes and risk of ischemic stroke: the Northern Manhattan Study. Stroke. 2012 May; 43(5): 1212–1217.

17. American Diabetes Association. Peripheral arterial disease in people with diabetes. Diabetes Care. 2003; 26(12): 3333–3341.

18. 2016 Alzheimer's disease facts and figures. Available from: http://www.alz.org/facts/. Accessed 2017 Feb 17.

19. De la Monte SM, Wands JR. Alzheimer's disease is type 3 diabetes—evidence reviewed. J Diabetes Sci Technol. 2008 Nov; 2(6): 1101–1113.

20. Barone BB, et al. Long-term all-cause mortality in cancer patients with preexisting diabetes mellitus: a systematic review and meta-analysis. JAMA. 2008 Dec 17; 300(23): 2754–2764.

21. Rinella ME. Nonalcoholic fatty liver disease: a systematic review. JAMA. 2015 Jun 9; 313(22): 2263–2273.

22. Ludwig E. [Urinary tract infections in diabetes mellitus.] Orv Hetil. 2008 Mar 30; 149(13): 597–600.

23. Pemayun TGD, et al. Risk factors for lower extremity amputation in patients with diabetic foot ulcers: a hospital-based case–control study. Diabetic Foot & Ankle. 2015; 6(1). doi: 10.3402/dfa.v6.29629. Accessed 2017 Jun 6.

24. Kahana M, et al. Skin tags: a cutaneous marker for diabetes mellitus. Acta Derm Venereol. 1987; 67(2): 175–177.

25. Lakin M, Wood H. Erectile dysfunction. Cleveland Clinic Center for Continuing Education. 2012 Nov. Available from: http://www.clevelandclinicmeded.com/medicalpubs/diseasemanagement/endocrinology/erectile-dysfunction/. Accessed 2017 Feb 17.

26. Sharpless JL. Polycystic ovary syndrome and the metabolic syndrome. Clinical Diabetes. 2003 Oct; 21(4): 154–161.

Chapter 4

1. Colditz GA, et al. Weight as a risk factor for clinical diabetes in women. Am J Epidemiol. 1990 Sep; 132(3): 501–513.

2. Powell A. Obesity? diabetes? we've been set up. Harvard Gazette. 2012 Mar 7. Available from: http://news.harvard.edu/gazette/story/2012/03/the-big-setup/. Accessed 2017 Jun 6.

3. Colditz GA, et al. Weight gain as a risk factor for clinical diabetes mellitus in women. Ann Intern Med. 1995 Apr 1; 122(7): 481–486.

4. Tobias DK, et al. Body-mass index and mortality among adults with incident type 2 diabetes. N Engl J Med. 2014; 370(3): 233–244.

5. Hu FB, et al. Diet, lifestyle, and the risk of type 2 diabetes mellitus in women. N Engl J Med. 2001; 345(11): 790–797.

6. Harcombe Z, et al. Evidence from randomised controlled trials did not support the introduction of dietary fat guidelines in 1977 and 1983: a systematic review and meta-analysis. Open Heart. 2015; 2(1): e000196. doi: 10.1136/openhrt-2014-000196. Accessed 2017 Jun 6.

7. Wei M, et al. Waist circumference as the best predictor of noninsulin dependent diabetes mellitus (NIDDM) compared to body mass index, waist/hip ratio and other anthropometric measurements in Mexican Americans—a 7-year prospective study. Obes Res. 1997 Jan; 5(1): 16–23.

8. McSweeny L. The devil inside. The Sydney Morning Herald. 2013 Sept 15. Available from: http://www.smh.com.au/lifestyle/the-devil-inside-20130910-2thyr.html. Accessed 2017 Jun 6.

9. Wildman RP. Healthy obesity. Curr Opin Clin Nutr Metab Care. 2009; 12(4): 438–443.

10. Ruderman N, et al. The metabolically obese, normal-weight individual revisited. Diabetes. 1998; 47(5): 699–713.

11. Taylor R, Holman RR. Normal-weight individuals who develop type 2 diabetes: the personal fat threshold. Clinical Science. 2015 Apr; 128(7): 405–410.

12. Després JP. Is visceral obesity the cause of the metabolic syndrome? Ann Med. 2006; 38(1): 52–63.

13. Taylor R, Holman RR. Normal-weight individuals who develop type 2 diabetes: the personal fat threshold. Clinical Science. 2015 Apr; 128(7): 405–410. Used with permission.

14. Matos LN, et al. Correlation of anthropometric indicators for identifying insulin sensitivity and resistance. Sao Paulo Med J. 2011; 129(1): 30–35.

15. Rexrode KM, et al. Abdominal adiposity and coronary heart disease in women. JAMA. 1998; 280(21): 1843–1848.

16. Wander PL, et al. Change in visceral adiposity independently predicts a greater risk of developing type 2 diabetes over 10 years in Japanese Americans. Diabetes Care. 2013; 36(2): 289–293.

17. Fujimoto WY, et al. Body size and shape changes and the risk of diabetes in the diabetes prevention program. Diabetes. 2007 Jun; 56(6): 1680–1685.

18. Klein S, et al. Absence of an effect of liposuction on insulin action and risk factors for coronary heart disease. N Engl J Med. 2004; 350(25): 2549–2557.

19. Ashwell M, et al. Waist-to-height ratio is more predictive of years of life lost than body mass index. PLoS One. 2014; 9(9): e103483. doi: 10.1371/journal. pone.0103483. Accessed 2017 Jun 6.

20. Ashwell M, et al. Waist-to-height ratio is more predictive of years of life lost than body mass index. PLoS One. 2014; 9(9): e103483. doi: 10.1371/journal. pone.0103483. Accessed 2017 Jun 6. Used with permission.

21. Bray GA, et al. Relation of central adiposity and body mass index to the development of diabetes in the Diabetes Prevention Program. Am J Clin Nutr. 2008; 87(5): 1212–1218; Fox CS, et al. Abdominal visceral and subcutaneous adipose tissue compartments: association with metabolic risk factors in the Framingham Heart Study. Circulation. 2007; 116(1): 39–48; Després JP. Intra-abdominal obesity: an untreated risk factor for type 2 diabetes and cardiovascular disease. J Endocrinol Invest. 2006; 2(3 Suppl): 77–82; Jakobsen MU, et al. Abdominal obesity and fatty liver. Epidemiol Rev. 2007; 29(1): 77–87.

22. Fabbrini E, Tamboli RA, et al. Surgical removal of omental fat does not improve insulin sensitivity and cardiovascular risk factors in obese adults. Gastroenterology. 2010; 139(2): 448–455.

23. Fabbrini E, et al. Intrahepatic fat, not visceral fat, is linked with metabolic complications of obesity. Proc Natl Acad Sci USA. 2009; 106(36): 15430–15435; Magkos F, Fabbrini E, et al. Increased whole-body adiposity without a concomitant increase in liver fat is not associated with augmented metabolic dysfunction. Obesity (Silver Spring). 2010; 18(8): 1510–1515.

24. Jakobsen MU, et al. Abdominal obesity and fatty liver. Epidemiol Rev. 2007; 29(1): 77–87.

25. Howard BV, et al. Low-fat dietary pattern and weight change over 7 years: the Women's Health Initiative Dietary Modification Trial. JAMA. 2006 Jan 4; 295(1): 39–49.

26. Fildes A, et al. Probability of an obese person attaining normal body weight: cohort study using electronic health records. Am J Public Health. 2015; 105(9): e54–e59.

Chapter 5

1. Banting W. Letter on Corpulence. Available from: http://www.thefitblog.net/ ebooks/LetterOnCorpulence/LetteronCorpulence.pdf. Accessed 2017 Jun 6.

Chapter 6

1. Pories WJ, et al. Surgical treatment of obesity and its effect on diabetes: 10-y follow-up. Am J Clin Nutr. 1992; 55(Suppl.): 582s–585s.

2. Based on data from Pories WJ, et al. Surgical treatment of obesity and its effect on diabetes: 10-y follow-up. Am J Clin Nutr. 1992 Feb; 55(2 Suppl): 582s–585s.

3. Insulinoma symptoms. Insulinoma Support Network. Available from: https:// insulinoma.co.uk/insulinoma-symptoms. Accessed 2017 Jun 6.

4. Tarchouli M, et al. Long-standing insulinoma: two case reports and review of the literature. BMC Res Notes. 2015; 8: 444.

5. Ghosh S, et al. Clearance of acanthosis nigricans associated with insulinoma following surgical resection. QJM. 2008 Nov; 101(11): 899–900. doi: 10.1093/qjmed/ hcn098. [Epub 2008 Jul 31.] Accessed 2017 Jun 6.

6. Rizza RA. Production of insulin resistance by hyperinsulinemia in man. Diabetologia. 1985; 28(2): 70–75.

7. Del Prato S. Effect of sustained physiologic hyperinsulinemia and hyperglycemia on insulin secretion and insulin sensitivity in man. Diabetologia. 1994 Oct; 37(10): 1025–1035.

8. Henry RR. Intensive conventional insulin therapy for type II diabetes. Diabetes Care. 1993; 16(1): 23–31.

9. Corkey BE, Banting lecture 2011: hyperinsulinemia: cause or consequence? Diabetes. 2012 Jan; 61(1): 4–13.

Chapter 7

1. Based on data from Tabák AG, et al. Trajectories of glycaemia, insulin sensitivity, and insulin secretion before diagnosis of type 2 diabetes: an analysis from the Whitehall II study. Lancet. 2009 Jun 27; 373(2682): 2215–2221.

2. Tabák AG, et al. Trajectories of glycaemia, insulin sensitivity, and insulin secretion before diagnosis of type 2 diabetes: an analysis from the Whitehall II study. Lancet. 2009 Jun 27; 373(2682): 2215–2221.

3. Weiss R, Taksali SE, et al. Predictors of changes in glucose tolerance status in obese youth. Diabetes Care. 2005; 28(4): 902–909.

4. Taksali SE, et al. High visceral and low abdominal subcutaneous fat stores in the obese adolescent: a determinant of an adverse metabolic phenotype. Diabetes. 2008; 57(2): 367–371.

5. Bawden S, et al. Increased liver fat and glycogen stores following high compared with low glycaemic index food: a randomized crossover study. Diabetes Obes Metab. 2017 Jan; 19(1): 70–77. doi: 10.1111/dom.12784. [Epub 2016 Sep 4]. Accessed 2017 Jun 6.

6. Suzuki A, et al. Chronological development of elevated aminotransferases in a non-alcoholic population. Hepatology. 2005; 41(1): 64–71.

7. Zelman S. The liver in obesity. AMA Arch Intern Med. 1952; 90(2): 141–156.

8. Ludwig J, et al. Nonalcoholic steatohepatitis: Mayo Clinic experiences with a hitherto unnamed disease. Mayo Clin Proc. 1980 Jul; 55(7): 434–438.

9. Leite NC, et al. Prevalence and associated factors of non-alcoholic fatty liver disease in patients with type-2 diabetes mellitus. Liver Int. 2009 Jan; 29(1): 113–119.

10. Seppala-Lindroos A, et al. Fat accumulation in the liver is associated with defects in insulin suppression of glucose production and serum free fatty acids independent of obesity in normal men. J Clin Endocrinol Metab. 2002 Jul; 87(7): 3023–3028.

11. Silverman JF, et al. Liver pathology in morbidly obese patients with and without diabetes. Am J Gastroenterol. 1990; 85(10): 1349–1355.

12. Fraser A, et al. Prevalence of elevated alanine-aminotransferase (ALT) among US adolescents and associated factors: NHANES 1999–2004. Gastroenterology. 2007; 133(6): 1814–1820.

13. Fabbrini E, et al. Intrahepatic fat, not visceral fat, is linked with metabolic complications of obesity. Proc Natl Acad Sci USA 2009; 106(36): 15430–15435; D'Adamo E, Caprio S. Type 2 diabetes in youth: epidemiology and pathophysiology. Diabetes Care. 2011; 34(Suppl 2): S161–S165.

14. Burgert TS, et al. Alanine aminotransferase levels and fatty liver in childhood obesity: associations with insulin resistance, adiponectin, and visceral fat. J Clin Endocrinol Metab. 2006; 91(11): 4287–4294.

15. Younossi AM, et al. Systematic review with meta-analysis: non-alcoholic steatohepatitis. Aliment Pharmacol Ther. 2014; 39(1): 3–14.

16. Angulo P. Nonalcoholic fatty liver disease. N Engl J Med. 2002; 346(16): 1221–1231.

17. Based on data from D'Adamo E, Caprio S. Type 2 diabetes in youth: epidemiology and pathophysiology. Diabetes Care. 2011 May; 34(Suppl 2): S161–S165.

18. Ryysy L, et al. Hepatic fat content and insulin action on free fatty acids and glucose metabolism rather than insulin absorption are associated with insulin requirements during insulin therapy in type 2 diabetic patients. Diabetes. 2000; 49(5): 749–758; 18.

19. Sevastianova K, et al. Effect of short-term carbohydrate overfeeding and long-term weight loss on liver fat in overweight humans. Am J Clin Nutr. 2012; 96(4): 727–734.

20. Schwarz JM, et al. Short-term alterations in carbohydrate energy intake in humans. Striking effects on hepatic glucose production, de novo lipogenesis, lipolysis, and whole-body fuel selection. J Clin Invest. 1995; 96(6): 2735–2743; Softic S, et al. Role of dietary fructose and hepatic de novo lipogenesis in fatty liver disease. Dig Dis Sci. 2016 May; 61(5): 1282–1293.

21. Chong MF, et al. Mechanisms for the acute effect of fructose on postprandial lipemia. Am J Clin Nutr. 2007; 85(6): 1511–1520.

22. Perseghin G. Reduced intrahepatic fat content is associated with increased whole-body lipid oxidation in patients with type 1 diabetes. Diabetologia. 2005; 48(12): 2615–2621.

23. Fabbrini E, et al. Intrahepatic fat, not visceral fat, is linked with metabolic complications of obesity. Proc Natl Acad Sci USA 2009; 106(36): 15430–15435.

24. Weiss R, Dufour S, et al. Pre-diabetes in obese youth: a syndrome of impaired glucose tolerance, severe insulin resistance, and altered myocellular and abdominal fat partitioning. Lancet. 2003; 362(9388): 951–957.

25. Kelley DE, et al. Skeletal muscle fatty acid metabolism in association with insulin resistance, obesity and weight loss. Am. J. Physiol Endocrinol Metab. 1999; 277(6 Pt 1): E1130–E1141.

26. Hue L, Taegtmeyer H. The Randle cycle revisited: a new head for an old hat. Am J Physiol Endocrinol Metab. 2009 Sep; 297(3): E578–E591.

27. Defronzo RA. Banting Lecture. From the triumvirate to the ominous octet: a new paradigm for the treatment of type 2 diabetes mellitus. Diabetes. 2009; 58(4): 773–795.

28. Taylor R. Type 2 diabetes: etiology and reversibility. Diabetes Care. 2013; 36(4): 1047–1055.

29. Mathur A, et al. Nonalcoholic fatty pancreas disease. HPB. 2007; 9(4): 312–318; Lee JS, et al. Clinical implications of fatty pancreas: Correlations between fatty pancreas and metabolic syndrome. World J Gastroenterol. 2009; 15(15): 1869–1875.

30. Ou HY, et al. The association between nonalcoholic fatty pancreas disease and diabetes. PLoS One. 2013; 8(5): e62561.

31. Steven S, et al. Weight loss decreases excess pancreatic triacylglycerol specifically in type 2 diabetes. Diabetes Care. 2016; 39(1): 158-165.

32. Heni M, et al. Pancreatic fat is negatively associated with insulin secretion in individuals with impaired fasting glucose and/or impaired glucose tolerance: a nuclear magnetic resonance study. Diabetes Metab Res Rev. 2010 Mar; 26(3): 200–205. doi: 10.1002/dmrr.1073; Tushuizen ME, et al. Pancreatic fat content and beta-cell function in men with and without type 2 diabetes. Diabetes Care. 2007; 30(11): 2916–2921.

33. Klein S, et al. Absence of an effect of liposuction on insulin action and risk factors for coronary heart disease. N Engl J Med. 2004; 350(25): 2549–2557.

34. Lim EL, et al. Reversal of type 2 diabetes: normalisation of beta cell function in association with decreased pancreas and liver triacylglycerol. Diabetologia. 2011; 54(10): 2506–2514.

35. Kim JY, et al. Obesity-associated improvements in metabolic profile through expansion of adipose tissue. J. Clin. Invest. 2007; 117(9): 2621–2637.

36. Rasouli N, et al. Ectopic fat accumulation and metabolic syndrome. Diabetes Obes Metab. 2007; 9(1): 1–10.

37. Vague J. The degree of masculine differentiation of obesities: a factor determining predisposition to diabetes, atherosclerosis, gout and uric calculous disease. Am J Clin Nutr. 1956; 4(1): 20–34.

38. Cao W, et al. Excess exposure to insulin is the primary cause of insulin resistance and its associated atherosclerosis. Curr Mol Pharmacol. 2011; 4(3): 154–166.

Chapter 8

1. Lustig, R. Sugar: the bitter truth. YouTube. Available from: https://www.youtube.com/watch?v=dBnniua6-oM. Accessed 2017 Jun 6.

2. Yudkin J. Pure, White and Deadly. London: HarperCollins; 1972.

3. Basu S, et al. The relationship of sugar to population-level diabetes prevalence: an econometric analysis of repeated cross-sectional data. PLoS One. 2013; 8(2): e57873.

4. Ridgeway, L. High fructose corn syrup linked to diabetes. USC News. 2012 Nov 28. Available from: https://news.usc.edu/44415/high-fructose-corn-syrup-linked-to-diabetes/. Accessed 2017 Jun 6.

5. Bizeau ME, Pagliassotti MJ. Hepatic adaptations to sucrose and fructose. Metabolism. 2005; 54(9): 1189–1201.

6. Faeh D, et al. Effect of fructose overfeeding and fish oil administration on hepatic de novo lipogenesis and insulin sensitivity in healthy men. Diabetes. 2005; 54(7): 1907–1913.

7. Lustig RH. Fructose: metabolic, hedonic, and societal parallels with ethanol. J Am Diet Assoc. 2010; 110(9): 1307–1321.

8. Yokoyama H, et al. Effects of excessive ethanol consumption on the diagnosis of the metabolic syndrome using its clinical diagnostic criteria. Intern Med. 2007; 46(17): 1345–1352.

9. Beck-Nielsen H, et al. Impaired cellular insulin binding and insulin sensitivity induced by high-fructose feeding in normal subjects. Am J Clin Nutr. 1980 Feb; 33(2): 273–278.

10. Stanhope KL, et al. Consuming fructose-sweetened, not glucose-sweetened, beverages increases visceral adiposity and lipids and decreases insulin sensitivity in overweight/obese humans. JCI. 2009; 119(5): 1322–1334.

11. Xu Y, et al. Prevalence and control of diabetes in Chinese adults. JAMA. 2013; 310(9): 948–959.

12. Zhou BF, et al. Nutrient intakes of middle-aged men and women in China, Japan, United Kingdom, and United States in the late 1990s: the INTERMAP study. J Hum Hypertens. (2003); 17(9): 623–630. doi: 10.1038/sj.jhh.1001605.

13. Based on data from Zhou BF, et al. Nutrient intakes of middle-aged men and women in China, Japan, United Kingdom, and United States in the late 1990s: the INTERMAP study. J Hum Hypertens. 2003 Sept; 17(9): 623–630. doi: 10.1038/sj. jhh.1001605. Accessed 2017 Jun 6.

14. Gross LS, et al. Increased consumption of refined carbohydrates and the epidemic of type 2 diabetes in the United States: an ecologic assessment. Am J Clin Nutr. 2004; 79(5): 774–779.

15. Basu S, et al. The relationship of sugar to population-level diabetes prevalence: an econometric analysis of repeated cross-sectional data. PLoS One. 2013; 8(2): e57873. doi: 10.1371/journal.pone.0057873. Accessed 2015 Apr 8.

16. Malik VS, et al. Sugar-sweetened beverages and risk of metabolic syndrome and type 2 diabetes. Diabetes Care. 2010; 33(11): 2477–2483.

17. Goran MI, et al. High fructose corn syrup and diabetes prevalence: A global perspective. Glob Pub Health. 2013; 8(1): 55–64.

18. Gross LS, et al. Increased consumption of carbohydrates and the epidemic of type 2 diabetes in the United States: an ecologic assessment. Am J Clin Nutr. 2004 May; 79(5): 774–779. Used with permission.

Chapter 9

1. Grundy SM, et al. Diagnosis and management of the metabolic syndrome: an American Heart Association/National Heart, Lung, and Blood Institute Scientific Statement. Circulation. 2005 Oct 25; 112(17): 2735–2752.

2. Ginsberg HN, MacCallum PR. The obesity, metabolic syndrome, and type 2 diabetes mellitus pandemic: Part I. increased cardiovascular disease risk and the importance of atherogenic dyslipidemia in persons with the metabolic syndrome and type 2 diabetes mellitus. Cardiometab Syndr. 2009 Spring; 4(2): 113–119.

3. Bremer AA, et al. Toward a unifying hypothesis of metabolic syndrome. Pediatrics. 2012; 129(3): 557–570.

4. Reaven GM. Banting lecture, 1988. Role of insulin resistance in human disease. Diabetes. 1988; 37(12): 1595–1607.

5. Ahrens EH, et al. Carbohydrate-induced and fat-induced lipemia. Trans. Assoc. Am. Phys. 1961; 74: 134–146.

6. Reaven GM, Calciano A, et al. Carbohydrate intolerance and hyperlipemia in patients with myocardial infarction without known diabetes mellitus. J Clin Endocrinol Metab. 1963; 23: 1013–1023.

7. Welborn TA, et al. Serum-insulin in essential hypertension and in peripheral vascular disease. Lancet. 1966; 1(7451): 1336–1337.

8. Lucas CP, et al. Insulin and blood pressure in obesity. Hypertension. 1985; 7: 702–706.

9. Huang PL. A comprehensive definition for metabolic syndrome. Dis Model Mech. 2009 May–Jun; 2(5–6): 231–237.

10. Reaven GM, et al. Insulin resistance as a predictor of age-related diseases. J Clin Endocrinol Metab. 2001; 86(8): 3574–3578; DeFronzo RA, Ferrannini E. Insulin resistance. A multifaceted syndrome responsible for NIDDM, obesity, hypertension, dyslipidemia, and atherosclerotic cardiovascular disease. Diabetes Care. 1991;14 (3): 173–194.

11. Lim JS, et al. The role of fructose in the pathogenesis of NAFLD and the metabolic syndrome. Nat Rev Gastroenterol Hepatol. 2010; 7(5): 251–264.

12. Grundy SM, et al. Transport of very low density lipoprotein triglycerides in varying degrees of obesity and hypertriglyceridemia. J. Clin. Invest. 1979; 63: 1274–1283.

13. Adiels M, et al. Overproduction of large VLDL particles is driven by increased liver fat content in man. Diabetologia. 2006; 49(4): 755–765.

14. Aarsland A, et al. Contributions of de novo synthesis of fatty acids to total

VLDL-triglyceride secretion during prolonged hyperglycemia/hyperinsulinemia in normal man. J Clin Invest. 1996; 98(9): 2008–2017.

15. Hiukka A, et al. Alterations of lipids and apolipoprotein CIII in VLDL subspecies in type 2 diabetes. Diabetologia. 2005; 48(6): 1207–1215; Grundy SM, et al. Transport of very low density lipoprotein triglycerides in varying degrees of obesity and hypertriglyceridemia. J. Clin. Invest. 1979; 63: 1274–1283.

16. Coulston AM, et al. Persistence of hypertriglyceridemic effects of low-fat, high-carbohydrate diets in NIDDM. Diabetes Care. 1989; 12(2): 94–100; Hyson DA, et al. Impact of dietary fat intake on postprandial lipemic response in postmenopausal women. FASEB J. 1999; 13: A213.

17. Reaven GM, et al. Role of insulin in endogenous hypertriglyceridemia. J Clin Invest. 1967; 46(11): 1756–1767; Stanhope KL, et al. Consumption of fructose and high fructose corn syrup increase postprandial triglycerides, LDL-cholesterol, and apolipoprotein-B in young men and women. J Clin Endocrinol Metab. 2011 Oct; 96(10): E1596–E1605.

18. Nordestgaard BG, et al. Nonfasting triglycerides and risk of myocardial infarction, ischemic heart disease, and death in men and women. JAMA. 2007; 298(3): 299–308.

19. Schwarz GG, et al. Fasting triglycerides predict recurrent ischemic events in patients with acute coronary syndrome treated with statins. J Am Coll Cardiol. 2015; 65(21): 2267–2275.

20. Miller M, et al. Triglycerides and cardiovascular disease: A scientific statement from the American Heart Association. Circulation. 2011; 123(20): 2292–2333.

21. HPS2-THRIVE Collaborative Group. Effects of extended-release niacin with laropiprant in high-risk patients. N Engl J Med. 2014; 371(3): 203–212; AIM-HIGH Investigators. Niacin in patients with low HDL cholesterol levels receiving intensive statin therapy. N Engl J Med. 2012; 365(24): 2255–2267.

22. Vergeer M, et al. The HDL hypothesis: does high-density lipoprotein protect from atherosclerosis? J Lipid Res. 2010 Aug; 51(8): 2058–2073.

23. Finelli C, et al. The improvement of large high-density lipoprotein (HDL) particle levels, and presumably HDL metabolism, depend on effect of low-carbohydrate diet and weight loss. EXCLI Journal. 2016; 15: 166–176.

24. ILLUMINATE Investigators. Effects of torcetrapib in patients at high risk for coronary events. N Engl J Med. 2007; 357(21): 2109–2122.

25. Ginsberg HN, et al. Regulation of plasma triglycerides in insulin resistance and diabetes. Arch Med Res. 2005; 36(3): 232–240.

26. Goodpaster BH, et al. Obesity, regional body fat distribution, and the metabolic syndrome in older men and women. Arch Intern Med. 2005; 165(7): 777–783.

27. Barzilai N, et al. Surgical removal of visceral fat reverses hepatic insulin resistance. Diabetes. 1999; 48(1): 94–98; Gabriely I, et al. Removal of visceral fat prevents insulin resistance and glucose intolerance of aging: an adipokine-mediated process? Diabetes. 2002; 51(10): 2951–2958.

28. Klein S, et al. Absence of an effect of liposuction on insulin action and risk factors for coronary heart disease. N Engl J Med. 2004; 350(25): 2549–2557.

29. Welborn T, et al. Serum-insulin in essential hypertension and in peripheral vascular disease. Lancet. 1966; 1(7451): 1336–1337.

30. Ferrannini E, et al. Insulin resistance, hyperinsulinemia, and blood pressure. Role of age and obesity. Hypertension. 1997; 30(5): 1144–1149.

31. Park SE, et al. Impact of hyperinsulinemia on the development of hypertension in normotensive, nondiabetic adults: a 4-year follow-up study. Metabolism. 2013 Apr; 62(4): 532–538.

32. Xun P, et al. Fasting insulin concentrations and incidence of hypertension, stroke, and coronary heart disease: a meta-analysis of prospective cohort studies. Am J Clin Nutr. 2013; 98(6): 1543–1554.

33. Christlieb R, et al. Is insulin the link between hypertension and obesity? Hypertension. 1985; 7(Suppl II): II-54–II-57; Cao W, et al. Excess exposure to insulin is the primary cause of insulin resistance and its associated atherosclerosis. Curr Mol Pharmacol. 2011; 4(3): 154–166.

34. Rieker RP, et al. Positive inotropic action of insulin on piglet heart. Yale. J. Biol. Med., 1975; 48: 353–360.

35. Bönner G. Hyperinsulinemia, insulin resistance, and hypertension. J Cardiovasc Pharmacol. 1994; 24(Suppl 2): S39–49.

36. Sattar N, et al. Serial metabolic measurements and conversion to type 2 diabetes in the West of Scotland Coronary Prevention Study. Diabetes. 2007; 56(4): 984–991.

37. Kolata G. Skinny and 119 pounds, but with the health hallmarks of obesity. New York Times. 2016 July 22. Available from: https://www.nytimes.com/2016/07/26/health/skinny-fat.html?mcubz=3

Chapter 10

1. Geller AI, et al. National estimates of insulin-related hypoglycemia and errors leading to emergency department visits and hospitalizations. JAMA Intern Med. 2014 May; 174(5): 678–686.

2. The Diabetes Control and Complications Trial Research Group. The effect of intensive treatment of diabetes on the development and progression of long-term complications in insulin-dependent diabetes mellitus. N Engl J Med. 1993; 329(14): 977–986.

3. The DCCT/EDIC Study Research Group. Intensive diabetes treatment and cardiovascular disease in patients with type 1 diabetes. N Engl J Med. 2005; 353(25): 2643–2653.

4. Based on data from The Diabetes Control and Complications Trial Research Group. Influence of intensive diabetes treatment on body weight and composition of adults with type 1 diabetes in the Diabetes Control and Complications Trial. Diabetes Care. 2001 Oct; 24(10): 1711–1721.

5. Purnell JQ, et al. The effect of excess weight gain with intensive diabetes treatment on cardiovascular disease risk factors and atherosclerosis in type 1 diabetes: Results from the Diabetes Control and Complications Trial / Epidemiology of Diabetes Interventions and Complications Study (DCCT/EDIC) study. Circulation. 2013 January 15; 127(2): 180–187. doi: 10.1161/CIRCULATIONAHA.111.077487. Accessed 2017 Jun 6.

6. Muis MJ. High cumulative insulin exposure: a risk factor of atherosclerosis in type 1 diabetes? Atherosclerosis. 2005 Jul; 181(1): 185–192.

7. UK Prospective Diabetes Study (UKPDS) Group. Intensive blood-glucose control with sulphonylureas or insulin compared with conventional treatment and risk of complications in patients with type 2 diabetes (UKPDS 33). Lancet. 1998 Sep 12; 352(9131): 837-53.

8. UK Prospective Diabetes Study (UKPDS) Group. Effect of intensive blood-glucose control with metformin on complications in overweight patients with type 2 diabetes (UKPDS 34). Lancet. 1998 Sep 12; 352(9131): 854-865.

9. Rosen CL, et al. The rosiglitazone story—lessons from an FDA Advisory Committee Meeting. N Engl J Med. 2007; 357(9): 844–846.

10. The ACCORD Study Group. Effects of intensive glucose lowering in type 2 diabetes. N Engl J Med. 2008 Jun 12; 358(24): 2545–2559.

11. The ADVANCE Collaborative Group. Intensive blood glucose control and vascular outcomes in patients with type 2 diabetes. N Engl J Med. 2008; 358(24): 2560–2572.

12. Duckworth W, et al. Glucose control and vascular complications in veterans with type 2 diabetes. N Engl J Med. 2009; 360(2): 129–139.

13. The ORIGIN Trial Investigators. Basal insulin and cardiovascular and other outcomes in dysglycemia. N Engl J Med. 2012; 367(4): 319–328.

14. The ACCORD Study Group. Long-term effects of intensive glucose lowering on cardiovascular outcome. N Engl J Med. 2011; 364(9): 818–828; Hayward RA, et al. Follow-up of glycemic control and cardiovascular outcomes in type 2 diabetes. N Engl J Med. 2015; 372(23): 2197–2206; Zoungas S, et al. Follow-up of blood-pressure lowering and glucose control in type 2 diabetes. N Engl J Med. 2014; 371(15): 1392–1406.

15. King P, et al. The UK Prospective Diabetes Study (UKPDS): clinical and therapeutic implications for type 2 diabetes. Br J Clin Pharmacol. 1999; 48(5): 643–648.

16. Soedamah-Muthu SS, et al. Relationship between risk factors and mortality in type 1 diabetic patients in Europe. The EURODIAB Prospective Complications Study (PCS). Diabetes Care. 2008; 31(7): 1360–1366.

17. Bain SC, et al. Characteristics of type 1 diabetes of over 50 years duration (the Golden Years Cohort). Diabetic Medicine. 2003; 20(10): 808–811.

18. Crofts CAP, et al. Hyperinsulinemia: a unifying theory of chronic disease? Diabesity. 2015; 1(4): 34–43; 41. Meinert CL, et al. A study of the effects of hypoglycemic agents on vascular complications in patients with adult-onset diabetes. II. Mortality results. Diabetes. 1970; 19(Suppl): 789–830.

19. Yudkin JS, et al. Intensified glucose lowering in type 2 diabetes: time for a reappraisal. Diabetologia. 2010 Oct; 53(10): 2079–2085.

20. Pradhan AD, et al. Effects of initiating insulin and metformin on glycemic control and inflammatory biomarkers among patients with type 2 diabetes The LANCET Randomized Trial. JAMA. 2009; 302(11): 1186–1194; Ridker PM, et al. C-reactive protein and other markers of inflammation in the prediction of cardiovascular disease in women. N Engl J Med. 2000; 342(12): 836–843.

21. Haffner SM, et al. Mortality from coronary heart disease in subjects with type 2 diabetes and in nondiabetic subjects with and without prior myocardial infarction. N Engl J Med, 1998; 339(4): 229–234.

22. Madonna R, De Caterina R. Prolonged exposure to high insulin impairs the endothelial PI3-kinase/Akt/nitric oxide signalling. Thromb Haemost. 2009; 101(2): 345–350; Okouchi M, et al. High insulin enhances neutrophil transendothelial migration through increasing surface expression of platelet endothelial cell adhesion molecule-1 via activation of mitogen activated protein kinase. Diabetologia. 2002; 45(10): 1449–1456; Pfeifle B, Ditschuneit H. Effect of insulin on growth of cultured human arterial smooth muscle cells. Diabetologia. 1981; 20(2): 155–158; Stout RW, et al. Effect of insulin on the proliferation of cultured primate arterial smooth muscle cells. Circ Res. 1975; 36: 319–327; Iida KT, et al. Insulin up-regulates tumor necrosis factor-alpha production in macrophages through

an extracellular-regulated kinase-dependent pathway. J Biol Chem. 2001; 276(35): 32531–32537.

23. Rensing KL. Endothelial insulin receptor expression in human atherosclerotic plaques: linking micro- and macrovascular disease in diabetes? Atherosclerosis. 2012; 222(1): 208–215.

24. Duff GL, McMillan GC. The effect of alloxan diabetes on experimental cholesterol atherosclerosis in the rabbit. J. Exp. Med. 1949; 89(6): 611–630.

25. Selvin E. Glycated hemoglobin, diabetes, and cardiovascular risk in nondiabetic adults. N Engl J Med. 2010; 362(9): 800–811.

26. Currie CJ, Poole CD, et al. Mortality and other important diabetes-related outcomes with insulin vs other antihyperglycemic therapies in type 2 diabetes. J Clin Endocrinol Metab. 2013; 98(2): 668–677.

27. Roumie CL, et al. Association between intensification of metformin treatment with insulin vs sulfonylureas and cardiovascular events and all-cause mortality among patients with diabetes. JAMA. 2014 Jun 11; 311(22): 2288–2296.

28. Currie CJ, Peters JR, et al. Survival as a function of HbA1c in people with type 2 diabetes: a retrospective cohort study. Lancet. 2010; 375(9713): 481–489.

29. Based on data from Gamble JM, et al. Insulin use and increased risk of mortality in type 2 diabetes. Diabetes, Obes Metab. 2010 Jan; 12(1): 47–53.

30. Després JP, et al. Hyperinsulinemia as an independent risk factor for ischemic heart disease. N Engl. J. Med. 1996; 334(15): 952–957.

31. Gamble JM, et al. Insulin use and increased risk of mortality in type 2 diabetes: a cohort study. Diabetes Obes Metab. 2010; 12(1): 47–53.

32. Margolis DJ, et al. Association between serious ischemic cardiac outcomes and medications used to treat diabetes. Pharmacoepidemiol Drug Saf. 2008 Aug; 17(8): 753–759.

33. Colayco DC, et al. A1C and cardiovascular outcomes in type 2 diabetes. Diabetes Care. 2011; 34(1): 77–83; In T2DM, lower HbA1c associated with elevated mortality risk vs moderate HbA1c | ADA. Univadis. 2016 Jun 13. Available from: http://www.univadis.com/viewarticle/in-t2dm-lower-hba1c-associated-with-elevated-mortality-risk-vs-moderate-hba1c-ada-414150. Accessed 2017 Jun 6.

34. Stoekenbroek RM, et al. High daily insulin exposure in patients with type 2 diabetes is associated with increased risk of cardiovascular events. Atherosclerosis. 2015 Jun; 240(2): 318–323.

35. Smooke S, et al. Insulin-treated diabetes is associated with a marked increase in mortality in patients with advanced heart failure. Am Heart J. 2005 Jan; 149(1): 168–174.

36. Johnson JA, Carstensen B, et al. Diabetes and cancer: evaluating the temporal relationship between type 2 diabetes and cancer incidence. Diabetologia. 2012; 55(6): 1607–1618.

37. Johnson JA, Gale EAM, et al. Diabetes, insulin use, and cancer risk: are observational studies part of the solution—or part of the problem? Diabetes. 2010 May; 59(5): 1129–1131.

38. Gunter MJ, Hoover DR, et al. Insulin, insulin-like growth factor-I, and risk of breast cancer in postmenopausal women. J Natl Cancer Inst. 2009; 101(1): 48–60.

39. Gunter MJ, Xie X, et al. Breast cancer risk in metabolically healthy but overweight postmenopausal women. Cancer Res. 2015; 75(2): 270–274.

40. Pal A, et al. PTEN mutations as a cause of constitutive insulin sensitivity and obesity. N Engl J Med. 2012; 367(11): 1002–1011.

41. Yang Y-X, et al. Insulin therapy and colorectal cancer risk among type 2 diabetes mellitus patients. Gastroenterology. 2004; 127(4): 1044–1050.

42. Currie CJ, Poole CD, Gale EA. The influence of glucose-lowering therapies on cancer risk in type 2 diabetes. Diabetologia. 2009; 52(9): 1766–1777.

43. Bowker SL, et al. Increased cancer-related mortality for patients with type 2 diabetes who use sulfonylureas or insulin. Diabetes Care. 2006 Feb; 29(2): 254–258.

Chapter 11

1. Menke A, et al. Prevalence of and trends in diabetes among adults in the United States, 1988–2012. JAMA. 2015; 314(10): 1021–1029.

2. Garber AJ, et al. Diagnosis and management of prediabetes in the continuum of hyperglycemia—when do the risks of diabetes begin? ACE/AACE Consensus Statement. Endocrine Practice. 2008 Oct; 14(7). Available from: https://www.aace.com/files/prediabetesconsensus.pdf. Accessed 2017 Jun 6.

3. Fauber J, et al. The slippery slope: a bittersweet diabetes economy. Medpage Today. 2014 Dec 21. Available from: http://www.medpagetoday.com/Cardiology/Diabetes/49227. Accessed 2017 Jun 6.

4. American Diabetes Association. Economic costs of diabetes in the U.S. in 2012. Diabetes Care. 2013 Apr; 36(4): 1033–1046.

5. Palmer E. The top 10 best-selling diabetes drugs of 2013. Fierce Pharma. 2014 Jun 17. Available from: http://www.fiercepharma.com/pharma/top-10-best-selling-diabetes-drugs-of-2013. Accessed 2017 Jun 6.

6. Based on data from Bianchi C, Del Prato S. Looking for new pharmacological treatments for type 2 diabetes. Diabetes Voice. 2011 Jun; 56: 28–31. Available from:

https://www.idf.org/e-library/diabetes-voice/issues/28-june-2011.html?lay-out=article&aid=65. Accessed 2017 Jun 14.

7. The ACCORD Study Group. Effects of intensive glucose lowering in type 2 diabetes. N Engl J Med. 2008; 358(24); 24: 2545–2559.

8. Centers for Disease Control and Prevention. Age-adjusted percentage of adults with diabetes using diabetes medication, by type of medication, United States, 1997–2011. 2012 Nov 20. Available from: http://www.cdc.gov/diabetes/statistics/meduse/fig2.htm. Accessed 2017 Jun 6.

9. Holman RR, et al. 10-year follow-up of intensive glucose control in type 2 diabetes. N Engl J Med. 2008 Oct; 359(15): 1577–1589.

10. Pantalone KM, et al. Increase in overall mortality risk in patients with type 2 diabetes receiving glipizide, glyburide or glimepiride monotherapy versus metformin: a retrospective analysis. Diabetes Obes Metab. 2012; 14(9): 803–809.

11. Tzoulaki I. Risk of cardiovascular disease and all cause mortality among patients with type 2 diabetes prescribed oral antidiabetes drugs. BMJ. 2009; 339: b4731.

12. Simpson SH, et al. Dose-response relation between sulfonylurea drugs and mortality in type 2 diabetes mellitus: a population-based cohort study. CMAJ. 2006; 174(2): 169–174.

13. Hong J, et al. Effects of metformin versus glipizide on cardiovascular outcomes in patients with type 2 diabetes and coronary artery disease. Diabetes Care. 2013 May; 36(5): 1304–1311.

14. Nissen SE, Wolski K. Effect of rosiglitazone on the risk of myocardial infarction and death from cardiovascular causes. N Engl J Med. 2007; 356(24): 2457–2471.

15. Rosen CL. The rosiglitazone story—lessons from an FDA Advisory Committee Meeting. N Engl J Med. 2007; 357: 844–846.

16. Rosen CL. Revisiting the rosiglitazone story—lessons learned. N Engl J Med. 2010; 363(9): 803–806.

17. Tuccori M, et al. Pioglitazone use and risk of bladder cancer: population based cohort study. BMJ. 2016; 352: i1541.

18. Scirica BM, et al. Saxagliptin and cardiovascular outcomes in patients with type 2 diabetes mellitus. N Engl J Med. 2013 Oct 3; 369(14): 1317–1326.

19. Green JB, et al. Effect of sitagliptin on cardiovascular outcomes in type 2 diabetes. N Engl J Med. 2015 Jul 16; 373(3): 232–242.

20. The world's top selling diabetes drugs. Pharmaceutical-technology.com. 2016 Mar 30. Available from: http://www.pharmaceutical-technology.com/features/featurethe-worlds-top-selling-diabetes-drugs-4852441/. Accessed 2017 Jan 31.

21. Rosenstock J, et al. Dual add-on therapy in type 2 diabetes poorly controlled with metformin monotherapy: a randomized double-blind trial of saxagliptin plus dapagliflozin addition versus single addition of saxagliptin or dapagliflozin to metformin. Diabetes Care. 2015 Mar; 38(3): 376-383.

22. Chilton RC, et al. Effects of empagliflozin on blood pressure and markers of arterial stiffness and vascular resistance in patients with type 2 diabetes. Diabetes Obes Metab. 2015 Dec; 17(12): 1180-1193.

23. Zinman B, et al. Empagliflozin, cardiovascular outcomes, and mortality in type 2 diabetes. N Engl J Med. 2015; 373(22): 2117–2128.

24. Wanner C, et al. Empaglifozin and progression of kidney disease in type 2 diabetes. N Engl J Med. 2016 Jul 28; 375(4): 323–334.

25. Blonde L, et al. Effects of canagliflozin on body weight and body composition in patients with type 2 diabetes over 104 weeks. Postgrad Med. 2016 May; 128(4): 371–380. doi: 10.1080/00325481.2016.1169894. Accessed 2017 Jun 6.

26. Wall JK. Analyst: Lilly's Jardiance diabetes pill could be a $6 billion-a-year blockbuster. Indianapolis Business Journal. 2015 Sep 21. Available from: http://www.ibj.com/blogs/12-the-dose/post/54957-analyst-lillys-jardiance-diabetes-pill-could-be-a-6-billion-a-year-blockbuster. Accessed 2017 Jun 6.

27. Chiasson JL, et al. Acarbose treatment and the risk of cardiovascular disease and hypertension in patients with impaired glucose tolerance. JAMA. 2003; 290(4): 486-494.

28. Marso SP et al. Liraglutide and cardiovascular outcomes in type 2 diabetes. N Engl J Med. 2016; 375(4): 311–322.

29. Erpeldinger S, et al. Efficacy and safety of insulin in type 2 diabetes: meta-analysis of randomised controlled trials. BMC Endocr Disord. 2016; 16(1): 39.

30. Palmer SC, et al. Comparison of clinical outcomes and adverse events associated with glucose-lowering drugs in patients with type 2 diabetes. A meta-analysis. JAMA. 2016; 316(3): 313–324.

31. Rodríguez-Gutiérrez R, Montori VM. Glycemic control for patients with type 2 diabetes mellitus: our evolving faith in the face of evidence. Circulation. 2016; 9(5): 504-512.

Chapter 12

1. Reversing type 2 diabetes starts with ignoring the guidelines. TEDxPerdueU. https://www.youtube.com/watch?v=da1vvigy5tQ. Accessed 2017 Jun 14.

2. Hallberg S, Hamdy O. Before you spend $26,000 on weight loss surgery, do this. The New York Times https://www.nytimes.com/2016/09/11/opinion/sunday/before-you-spend-26000-on-weight-loss-surgery-do-this.html?_r=0. Accessed 2017 Jun 14.

3. Kolata G. Diabetes and your diet: the low-carb debate. The New York Times. 2016 Sep 16. Available from: http://www.nytimes.com/2016/09/16/health/type-2-diabetes-low-carb-diet.html. Accessed 2017 Jun 6.

4. Nutrition recommendations and interventions for diabetes: a position statement of the American Diabetes Association. Diabetes Care. 2008; 31(Suppl 1): s61–s78.

5. TODAY Study Group. A clinical trial to maintain glycemic control in youth with type 2 diabetes. N Engl J Med. 2012; 366(24): 2247–2256.

6. Hu FB, et al. Dietary fat intake and the risk of coronary heart disease in women. N Engl J Med. 1997; 337(21): 1491–1499.

7. Howard BV, Van Horn L, et al. Low-fat dietary pattern and risk of cardiovascular disease: the Women's Health Initiative Randomized Controlled Dietary Modification Trial. JAMA. 2006 Feb 8; 295(6): 655–666.

8. Howard BV, Manson JE, et al. Low-fat dietary pattern and weight change over 7 years: the Women's Health Initiative Dietary Modification Trial. JAMA. 2006 Jan 4; 295(1): 39–49.

9. Oglesby P, et al. A longitudinal study of coronary heart disease. Circulation. 1963; 28: 20–31; Morris JN, et al. Diet and heart: a postscript. BMJ. 1977; 2(6098): 1307–1314; Yano K, et al. Dietary intake and the risk of coronary heart disease in Japanese men living in Hawaii. Am J Clin Nutr. 1978; 31(7): 1270–1279; Garcia-Palmieri MR, et al. Relationship of dietary intake to subsequent coronary heart disease incidence: The Puerto Rico Heart Health Program. Am J Clin Nutr. 1980; 33(8): 1818–1827; Shekelle RB, et al. Diet, serum cholesterol, and death from coronary disease: the Western Electric Study. N Engl J Med. 1981; 304(2): 65–70.

10. Mente A, et al. A systematic review of the evidence supporting a causal link between dietary factors and coronary heart disease. Arch Intern Med. 2009; 169(7): 659–669.

11. Wing R, et al. Cardiovascular effects of intensive lifestyle intervention in type 2 diabetes. N Engl J Med. 2013; 369(2): 145–154.

12. Park A. Where dietary-fat guidelines went wrong. Time. 2015 Feb 9. Available from: http://time.com/3702058/dietary-guidelines-fat-wrong/. Accessed 2017 Jun 6.

13. Booth FW, et al. Waging war on physical inactivity: using modern molecular ammunition against an ancient enemy. J Appl Physiol 2002; 93(1): 3–30.

14. O'Gorman DJ, Krook A. Exercise and the treatment of diabetes and obesity. Med Clin N Am. 2011; 95(5): 953–969.

15. O'Gorman DJ, Karlsson HKR, et al. Exercise training increases insulin-stimulated glucose disposal and GLUT4 (SLC2A4) protein content in patients with type 2 diabetes. Diabetologia. 2006; 49(12): 2983–2992.

16. Boulé NG, et al. Effects of exercise on glycemic control and body mass in type 2 diabetes mellitus. JAMA. 2001; 286(10): 1218–1227.

Chapter 13

1. Moore T. Experts urge surgery to cure type-2 diabetes. SkyNews. 2016 May 24. Available from: http://news.sky.com/story/experts-urge-surgery-to-cure-type-2-diabetes-10293295. Accessed 2017 Jun 6.

2. Moshiri M, et al. Evolution of bariatric surgery: a historical perspective. Am J Roentgenol. 2013 Jul; 201(1): W40–48.

3. Rubino F. Medical research: Time to think differently about diabetes. Nature. 2016 May 24. Available from: http://www.nature.com/news/medical-research-time-to-think-differently-about-diabetes-1.19955. Accessed 2017 Jun 6.

4. Kolata G. After weight-loss surgery, a year of joys and disappointments. The New York Times. 2016 Dec 27. Available from: https://www.nytimes.com/2016/12/27/health/bariatric-surgery.html. Accessed 2017 Jun 6.

5. Keidar A, et al. Long-term metabolic effects of laparoscopic sleeve gastrectomy. JAMA Surg. 2015 Nov; 150(11): 1051–1057.

6. Based on data from Schauer PR, et al. Bariatric surgery versus intensive medical therapy in obese patients with diabetes. N Engl J Med. 2012 Apr 26; 366(17): 1567–1576.

7. Schauer PR, et al. Bariatric surgery versus intensive medical therapy in obese patients with diabetes. N Engl J Med. 2012 Apr 26; 366(17): 1567–1576.

8. Inge TH, et al. Weight loss and health status 3 years after bariatric surgery in adolescents. N Engl J Med. 2016; 374(2): 113–123.

9. Pories WJ, et al. Surgical treatment of obesity and its effect on diabetes: 10-y follow-up. Am J Clin Nutr. 1992 Feb; 55(2 Suppl): 582s–585s.

10. American Diabetes Association. Consensus from diabetes organizations worldwide: metabolic surgery recognized as a standard treatment option for type 2 diabetes. 2016 May 24. Available from: http://www.diabetes.org/newsroom/press-releases/2016/consensus-from-diabetes-organizations-worldwide-metabolic-surgery-recognized-as-a-standard-treatment-option-for-type-2-diabetes.html. Accessed 2017 Jun 6.

11. Klein S, et al. Absence of an effect of liposuction on insulin action and risk factors for coronary heart disease. N Engl J Med. 2004; 350(25): 2549–2557.

12. Hallberg S, Hamdy O. Before you spend $26,000 on weight-loss surgery, do this. The New York Times. 2016 Sep 10. Available from: https://www.nytimes.com/2016/09/11/opinion/sunday/before-you-spend-26000-on-weight-loss-surgery-do-this.html?_r=0. Accessed 2017 Jun 6.

Chapter 14

1. Knapton S. Obese three-year-old becomes youngest child diagnosed with Type 2 diabetes. The Telegraph. 2015 Sep 17. Available from: http://www.telegraph.co.uk/news/health/news/11869249/Obese-three-year-old-becomes-youngest-child-diagnosed-with-Type-2-diabetes.html. Accessed 2017 Jun 6.

2. World Health Organization. Global report on diabetes. 2016. Available from: http://www.who.int/diabetes/global-report/en/. Accessed 2017 Jun 6.

3. American Diabetes Association. Standards of medical care in diabetes 2016. Diabetes Care. 2016 Jan; 39(Suppl 1): S25–26.

4. American Diabetes Association. Nutrition recommendations and interventions for diabetes. A position statement of the American Diabetes Association. Diabetes Care. 2008 Jan; 31(Suppl 1): S61–S78.

5. De Lorgeril M, et al. Mediterranean diet, traditional risk factors, and the rate of cardiovascular complications after myocardial infarction: final report of the Lyon Diet Heart Study. Circulation. 1999; 99(6): 779–785.

6. Mozzafarian D, Rimm EB, et al. Dietary fats, carbohydrate, and progression of coronary atherosclerosis in postmenopausal women. Am J Clin Nutr. 2004; 80(5): 1175–1184.

7. Estruch R, et al. Primary prevention of cardiovascular disease with a Mediterranean diet. N Engl J Med. 2013 Apr 4; 368(14): 1279–1290.

8. Hoenselaar R. Further response from Hoenselaar. Br J Nutr. 2012 Sep; 108(5): 939–942.

9. Siri-Tarino PW, et al. Meta-analysis of prospective cohort studies evaluating the association of saturated fat with cardiovascular disease. Am J Clin Nutr. 2010; 91(3); 535–546.

10. Kagan A, et al. Dietary and other risk factors for stroke in Hawaiian Japanese men. 1985; 16(3): 390–396; Gillman MW, et al. Inverse association of dietary fat with development of ischemic stroke in men. JAMA. 1997 Dec 24–31; 278(24): 2145–2150.

11. Based on data from Yamagishi K, et al. Dietary intake of saturated fatty acids and mortality from cardiovascular diseases in Japanese: the Japan Collaborative Cohort Study for Evaluation of Cancer Risk (JACC) study. Am J Clin Nutr. 2009 Oct; 92(4): 759-765. Available from: doi:10.3945/ajcn.2009.29146. Accessed 2017 Jun 6.

12. Hu FB, Stampfer MJ, et al. Frequent nut consumption and risk of coronary heart disease in women: prospective cohort study. BMJ. 1998; 317(7169): 1341–1345.

13. Burr ML. Effects of changes in fat, fish, and fibre intakes on death and myocardial reinfarction: diet and reinfarction trial (DART). Lancet. 1989 Sep 30; 2(8666): 757–756.

14. Mozaffarian D, Cao H, et al. Trans-palmitoleic acid, metabolic risk factors, and new-onset diabetes in US adults. Ann Intern Med. 2010 December 21; 153(12): 790–799.

15. Liu L, et al. Egg consumption and risk of coronary heart disease and stroke: dose-response meta-analysis of prospective cohort studies. BMJ. 2013 Jan 7; 346: e8539.

16. Shin JY, et al. Egg consumption in relation to risk of cardiovascular disease and diabetes. Am J Clin Nutr. 2013 July; 98(1): 146–159.

17. Masharani U, et al. Metabolic and physiologic effects from consuming a hunter-gatherer (Paleolithic)-type diet in type 2 diabetes. European J Clin Nutr. 2105; 69(8): 944–948.

18. Hu FB, Manson JE, et al. Types of dietary fat and risk of coronary heart disease: a critical review. J Am Coll Nutr. 2001; 20(1): 5–19.

19. Liu S, et al. A prospective study of dietary glycemic load, carbohydrate intake, and risk of coronary heart disease in US women. Am J Clin Nutr. 2000 Jun; 71(6): 1455–1461.

20. Based on data from Liu S, et al. A prospective study of dietary glycemic load, carbohydrate intake, and risk of coronary heart disease in US women. Am J Clin Nutr. 2000 Jun; 71(6): 1455–1461.

21. Ajala O, et al. Systematic review and meta-analysis of different dietary approaches to the management of type 2 diabetes. Am J Clin Nutr. 2013; 97(3): 505–516.

22. Goday A, et al. Short-term safety, tolerability and efficacy of a very low-calorie-ketogenic diet interventional weight loss program versus hypocaloric diet in patients with type 2 diabetes mellitus. Nutrition & Diabetes. 2016; 6: e230.

23. Based on data from Cohen E, et al. Statistical review of US macronutrient consumption data, 1965–2011: Americans have been following dietary guidelines, coincident with the rise in obesity. Nutrition. 2015 May; 31(5): 727–732.

24. Centers for Disease Control and Prevention. Trends in intake of energy and macro-nutrients—United States: 1971 to 2000. JAMA. 2004; 291: 1193–1194.

25. Villegas R, et al. Prospective study of dietary carbohydrates, glycemic index, glycemic load, and incidence of type 2 diabetes mellitus in middle-aged Chinese women. Arch Intern Med. 2007 Nov 26; 167(21): 2310–2316.

26. Based on data from Harvard Medical School. Glycemic index and glycemic load for 100+ foods: measuring carbohydrate effects can help glucose management. Harvard Health Publications [Internet]. February 2015. Updated 27 August 2015. Available from: http://www.health.harvard.edu/diseases-and-conditions/glycemic_index_and_glycemic_load_for_100_foods. Accessed 2017 Jun 6.

27. Trowell HC, Burkitt DP. Western diseases: their emergence and prevention. Boston: Harvard University Press; 1981.

28. Lindeberg S, et al. Low serum insulin in traditional Pacific Islanders—the Kitava study. Metabolism. 1999 Oct; 48(10): 1216–1219.

29. Giugliano D, et al. Effects of a Mediterranean-style diet on the need for antihyperglycemic drug therapy in patients with newly diagnosed type 2 diabetes. Ann Int Med. 2009 Sep 1; 151(5): 306–313.

30. Feinman RD, et al. Dietary carbohydrate restriction as the first approach in diabetes management: Critical review and evidence base. Nutrition. 2015; 31(1): 1–13.

31. Banting W. Letter on Corpulence. Available from: http://www.thefitblog.net/ebooks/LetterOnCorpulence/LetteronCorpulence.pdf. Accessed 2017 Jun 6.

32. Unwin DJ, et al. It's the glycaemic response to, not the carbohydrate content of food that matters in diabetes and obesity: The glycaemic index revisited. Journal of Insulin Resistance. 2016; 1(1). Available from: http://www.insulinresistance.org/index.php/jir/article/view/8. Accessed 2017 Jun 14. Used with permission.

33. Hughes T, Davies M. Thousands of diabetics adopt high-protein low-carb diet in backlash against official NHS eating plan. The Daily Mail. 2016 May 31. http://www.dailymail.co.uk/news/article-3617076/Diabetes-patients-defy-NHS-Thousands-rebel-against-guidelines-controlling-condition-diet-low-carbohydrates.html. Accessed 2017 Jun 12.

34. Hamdy O. Nutrition revolution—the end of the high carbohydrates era for diabetes prevention and management. US Endocrinology. 2014; 10(2): 103–104.

35. Third national health and nutrition examination survey. Medscape J Med. 2008; 10(7): 160.

36. Siri-Tarino PW, et al., Meta-analysis of prospective cohort studies evaluating the association of saturated fat with cardiovascular disease. Am J Clin Nutr. 2010;

91(3): 535–546; Estruch R, et al. Primary prevention of cardiovascular disease with a Mediterranean diet. N Engl J Med. 2013 Apr 4; 368(14): 1279–1290.

Chapter 15

1. Lingvay I. Rapid improvement of diabetes after gastric bypass surgery: is it the diet or the surgery? Diabetes Care. 2013 Sep; 36(9): 2741–2747.

2. American Diabetes Association. Standards of medical care in diabetes 2016. Diabetes Care. 2016; 39(Suppl 1): S48.

3. Fildes A, et al. Probability of an obese person attaining normal body weight: cohort study using electronic health records. Am J Public Health. 2015; 105(9): e54–e59.

4. Harvie MN, et al. The effects of intermittent or continuous energy restriction on weight loss and metabolic disease risk markers: a randomized trial in young overweight women. Int J Obes (Lond). 2011 May; 35(5): 714–727.

5. Based on data from Harvie MN, et al. The effect of intermittent or continuous energy restriction on weight loss and metabolic disease risk markers: A randomized trial in young overweight women. Int J Obes. 2011 May; 35(5): 714–727.

6. Catenacci VA, et al. A randomized pilot study comparing zero-calorie alternate-day fasting to daily caloric restriction in adults with obesity. Obesity (Silver Spring). 2016 Sep; 24(9): 1874–1883.

7. Johannsen DL, et al. Metabolic slowing with massive weight loss despite preservation of fat-free mass. J Clin Endocrinol Metab. 2012 Jul; 97(7): 2489–2496.

8. Best fast weight-loss diets. U.S. News & World Report. Available from: http://health.usnews.com/best-diet/best-fast-weight-loss-diets. Accessed 2017 Feb 3.

9. Callahan M. "We're all fat again": More "Biggest Loser" contestants reveal secrets. New York Post. 2015 Jan 25. Available from: http://nypost.com/2015/01/25/were-all-fat-again-more-biggest-loser-contestants-reveal-secrets/. Accessed 2017 Jun 6.

10. Fothergill E, et al. Persistent metabolic adaptation 6 years after "The Biggest Loser" competition. Obesity. 2016; 24(8): 1612–1619.

11. Keys A, et al. The Biology of Human Starvation. 2 vols. St. Paul, MN: University of Minnesota Press; 1950.

12. Zauner C, et al. Resting energy expenditure in short-term starvation is increased as a result of an increase in serum norepinephrine. Am J Clin Nutr. 2000; 71(6): 1511–1515.

13. Heilbronn LK, et al. Alternate-day fasting in nonobese subjects: effects on body weight, body composition, and energy metabolism. Am J Clin Nutr. 2005; 81(1): 69–73.

14. Based on data from Zauner C. Resting energy expenditure in short-term starvation is increased as a result of an increase in serum norepinephrine. Am J Clin Nutr. 2000 Jun; 71(6): 1511–1515.

15. Nuttall FQ, et al. Comparison of a carbohydrate-free diet vs. fasting on plasma glucose, insulin and glucagon in type 2 diabetes. Metabolism. 2015 Feb; 64(2): 253–262.

16. Jackson I, et al. Effect of fasting on glucose and insulin metabolism of obese patients. Lancet. 1969; 293(7589): 285–287.

17. Li G, et al. The long-term effect of lifestyle interventions to prevent diabetes in the China Da Qing Diabetes Prevention Study: A 20-year follow-up study. Lancet. 2008; 371(9626): 1783–1789.

18. Wareham NJ. The long-term benefits of lifestyle interventions for prevention of diabetes. Lancet Diabetes & Endocrinology. 2014 Jun; 2(6): 441–442.

19. Diabetes Prevention Program Research Group. Reduction in the incidence of type 2 diabetes with lifestyle intervention or metformin. N Engl J Med. 2002; 346(6): 393–403.

20. Diabetes Prevention Program Research Group. 10-year follow-up of diabetes incidence and weight loss in the Diabetes Prevention Program Outcomes Study. Lancet. 2009; 374(9702): 1677–1686.

21. Ramachandran A, et al. The Indian Diabetes Prevention Programme shows that lifestyle modification and metformin prevent type 2 diabetes in Asian Indian subjects with impaired glucose tolerance (IDPP-1). Diabetologia. 2006; 49(2): 289–297.

22. Tuomilehto J, et al. Prevention of type 2 diabetes mellitus by changes in lifestyle among subjects with impaired glucose tolerance. N Engl J Med. 2001; 344(18): 1343–1350.

23. Kosaka K, et al. Prevention of type 2 diabetes by lifestyle intervention: a Japanese trial in IGT males. Diabetes Res Clin Pract. 2005; 67(2): 152–162.

Afterword

1. Fung, Jason. "The Aetiology of Obesity." YouTube. Available from: https://www.youtube.com/watch?v=YpllomiDMX0.

2. Fung, Jason. "Intensive Dietary Management." Available from: www.IDMprogram.com.

INDEX

....

Figures and tables indicated by page numbers in italics

insulin resistance and, 44, 80, 82,
83, 91; metabolic syndrome and,
116; non-alcoholic fatty liver
disease (NAFLD), 29–30, 81–83;
non-alcoholic steatohepatitis
(NASH), 30, 44, 82; prevalence,
82–83; related diseases, 82;
reversibility of, 84; from sucrose,
186
fatty muscle, 85–86, 91
fatty pancreas, 89–90, 91
feet: nerve damage, 25–26; non-
healing foot ulcers, 28, 30, 72
Finland, 205
fish, 177
Fleming, Alexander, 61
fois gras, 84–85
food pyramid, 9, *10*, 152
food rationing, 191
food storage. *See* de novo lipogenesis
(DNL); glycogen
foregut hypothesis, 170
Framingham studies, 27, 111
French paradox, 176
Fröhlich, Alfred, 81
fructose: consumption increases,
97–98; de novo lipogenesis
(DNL) from, 109; elimination
from diet, 185–86; fatty liver
role, 84, 99, 104, 186; hypertriglyceridemia from, 110–11;
insulin resistance from, 100–101,
182; metabolism of, 96, 98–99,
103–4; molecular structure, 95;
sources, 96, 97, *185*; toxicity and
health risks, 97, 98, 102–3, 103–4,
181. *See also* high-fructose corn
syrup; sugar
fruit, 40, 96, 97, 186

Fung, Jason, 211–12, 214–15
fungal infections, 30, 31

gastric dumping syndrome, 166, 167
gastric "lap" band, 167
gestational diabetes, 14
ghrelin, 48, 170
glicizide, 141
glipizide, 141
Global Report on Diabetes (WHO), 175
glucagon, 203
glucagon-like peptide 1 (GLP-1) analogs, 148, 149
gluconeogenesis, 52, 54, 87, 144
glucose: metabolism of, 18, 98, 104;
molecular structure, 95. *See also*
blood glucose; hyperglycemia;
hypoglycemia
glucotoxicity: acarbose and, 147;
cancer and, 136; DPP-4 inhibitors and, 145; GLP-1 analogs
and, 148; medication overview,
148–49; replacement with insulin toxicity, 125–26, 130–31, 134,
136; SGLT2 inhibitors and, 146;
sulfonylureas (SUs) and, 141;
type 1 diabetes and, 124–25, 126;
type 2 diabetes and, 126–29, 141
glyburide, 141
glycemic index, 40, 96, 97
glycemic load, 40, 178, *180*
glycogen: creation and storage in
liver, 51, 79, 98, 104, 109; energy
produced from, 52; fasting usage
of, 52, 171, 198; in muscles, 51, 85
Golden Years Cohort Study, 130
Greek Orthodox Church, 72
Gregory the Great, 190
growth hormone, 49, 64, 197, 203

hypertension (high blood pressure),
106, 107, 114–15, 147
hypertriglyceridemia, 107, 109–11
hypoglycemia: biguanide drugs
and, 144; complications from,
123–24; DPP-4 inhibitors and,
145; elevated glucose levels to
avoid, 124; insulinomas and, 59;
intensive insulin treatment and,
125; medication during fasting
and, 200, 201
hypothalamic area, brain, 81

incretins, 144–45, 148, 170
India, 3, 205
infections, 30–31
insulin: carbohydrate-insulin
hypothesis, 54–55; as conventional diabetes treatment, 123;
discovery of, 5, 7; dosage issues,
123–24; energy storage-and-release role, 18, 49, 50–53, 108–9;
failure to cure type 2 diabetes,
126–29, 140, 148, 150, 206, 212;
fasting insulin, 57, 58, 65, 169,
194; health costs from, 139;
hypoglycemia from, 200; production by pancreas, 49; type 1
diabetes benefit, 124–25; weight
gain from, xiv–xv, 53–54, 125,
127, 129. *See also* hyperinsulinemia; insulin resistance
insulin-dependent diabetes, 8
insulinoma, 53–54, 59
insulin resistance: introduction,
20, 77; abdominal (visceral)
fat role, 79, 90; beta cell dysfunction from, 78; caused by
hyperinsulinemia, 56, 63, 64–65,
68, 69–70; de novo lipogenesis

(DNL) and, 67, 70; emergence
timeline prior to type 2 diabetes, 79; erectile dysfunction
and, 31; fatty liver role, 80, 83;
fatty muscle role, 86; fructose role, 100–101, 182; high
fasting insulin from, 65; intermittent fasting on, 194–95;
lock-and-key paradigm, 66,
68; obesity and, 57–58; overflow phenomenon, xvi–xviii,
68–71, 171; polycystic ovarian
syndrome (PCOS) and, 32; as
protective mechanism, 58–59,
113, 117; Randle cycle and, 87;
reversibility of, 59–60. *See also*
hyperinsulinemia
Intensive Dietary Management program, 201–2, 216
INTERMAP study, 101
intermittent fasting. *See* fasting,
intermittent
International Diabetes Federation,
11, 169
intrahepatic fat, 44. *See also* fatty
liver
intramyocyte lipid accumulation, 85.
See also fatty muscle
intra-organic fat, 44. *See also* fat,
abdominal
iron supplements, 201

Japan, 10, 69, 176, 205
jejunocolic bypass surgery, 164–65
jejunoileal bypass surgery, 165
Jenner, Edward, 62
Joslin, Elliott, 5, 6–7, 8, 184, 190, 199
juvenile diabetes, 8, 18. *See also* type
1 diabetes

Kahn, Richard, 152
ketoacidosis, diabetic, 15–16, 124, 146
Keys, Ancel, 94, 196
kidney disease (nephropathy), 23–25
kidney infection, 30, 146
Kitava (island), 180

lactic acidosis, 144
Lana (case study), 209
Lantus, 139, 145
LCHF (low-carbohydrate, healthy-fat) diet, 40, 187–88, 191, 198–99, 215, 216
LDL (low-density lipoprotein), 108, 111
LEADER trial, 148
lean mass, 195, 197
leptin, 112–13
lipodystrophy, 116–17
lipoprotein lipase (LPL), 53, 111
Liraglutide, 148
liver, 108–9. *See also* fatty liver
lock-and-key paradigm, 66, 68
LookAHEAD (Action for Health in Diabetes) trial, 154–55
low-carbohydrate, healthy-fat· (LCHF) diet, 40, 187–88, 191, 198–99, 215, 216
low-carbohydrate diets, 4, 55, 174, 178–79, 181, 182–85
low-density lipoprotein (LDL), 108, 111
low-fat diets, 9, 40, 151, 152–53, 175–76. *See also* fat, dietary
low glycemic-index diet, 178–79
LPL (lipoprotein lipase), 53, 111
Ludwig, Jürgen, 81, 82
Lustig, Robert, 94, 103, 105

Lyon Diet Heart Study, 175

Macleod, John, 7
macronutrients, 50. *See also* carbohydrates; fat, dietary; protein
macrovascular diseases, 26–29; introduction, 22; atherosclerosis, 26–27; heart disease, 27–28; peripheral vascular disease (PVD), 28–29; stroke, 28. *See also* cardiovascular (heart) disease
madhumeha (honey urine), 3
magnesium supplements, 201
marbling, 86
medication: donations from pharmaceutical companies, 138–39; failure of, xv, xviii, 126–29, 148–50, 212; fasting and, 200–201; health costs from, 139; increase in types, 139; popularity despite lack of evidence, 138, 150; revenue from, 139
medication, specific types: overview, 149; acarbose, 147, 149; alpha-glucosidase inhibitors, 147; biguanide drugs, 144; dipeptidyl peptidase-4 (DPP-4) inhibitors, 144–45, 149, 150, 200; glucagon-like peptide 1 (GLP-1) analogs, 148, 149; insulin, 139, 140, 148, 150; metformin, 54, 127, 129, 143–44, 149, 200, 201; pioglitazone (Actos), 142, 143; rosiglitazone (Avandia), 142–43; sitagliptin, 145; sodium-glucose cotransporter 2 (SGLT2), 145–46, 149, 200; sulfonylureas (SUs), 54, 126, 128, 129, 141–42, 148, 200;